Plant Based Diet Cookbook

Delicious Vegan Recipes for Busy People, Ready in Thirty Minutes. Quick and Easy Vegetarian Meals for Healthy Eating To Prevent And Cure Disease And Energize Your Body.

Table of Contents

Introduction 1

Chapter 1.   Breakfast Recipes 3

Vegan Breakfast Sandwich...3

Vegan Fried Egg 4

Sweet Crepes..5

Spinach Artichoke Quiche...6

Tofu Scramble..7

Pumpkin Muffins..8

Tomato and Asparagus Quiche...10

Simple Vegan Breakfast Hash 12

Chickpeas On Toast...13

Blueberry Muffins..14

Ultimate Breakfast Sandwich..15

Waffles with Fruits 16

Chickpea Omelet..17

Scrambled Tofu Breakfast Burrito 18

Pancake..20

Chapter 2.   Lunch Recipes...21

Cashew Siam Salad..21

Avocado and Cauliflower Hummus...22

Raw Zoodles with Avocado 'N Nuts 23

Cauliflower Sushi...24

Spinach and Mashed Tofu Salad 25

Cucumber Edamame Salad...26

Artichoke White Bean Sandwich Spread 27

Buffalo Chickpea Wraps...28

Coconut Veggie Wraps 29

Cucumber Avocado Sandwich 30

Lentil Sandwich Spread 31

Mediterranean Tortilla Pinwheels..32

Rice and Bean Burritos 33

Ricotta Basil Pinwheels 34

Delicious Sloppy Joes With No Meat 35

Spicy Hummus and Apple Wrap 36

Sun-dried Tomato Spread...37

Sweet Potato Sandwich Spread 38

Zucchini Sandwich with Balsamic Dressing 39

Chapter 3.   Soup Recipes...**40**

    Butternut Squash and Coconut Milk Soup 40

    Broccoli Cheese Soup 42

    Potato and Kale Soup 43

    Vegan Pho 44

    Roasted Cauliflower Soup 45

    Curried Apple and Sweet Potato Soup 47

    Ramen Noodle Soup 49

    Lasagna Soup 51

    Hot and Sour Soup 53

    Potato and Corn Chowder 55

    Thai Coconut Soup 56

    Spanish Chickpea and Sweet Potato Stew 57

    Pomegranate and Walnut Stew 59

    Sweet Potato, Kale and Peanut Stew 60

    Vegetarian Irish Stew 62

    White Bean and Cabbage Stew 63

    Spinach and Cannellini Bean Stew 64

    Fennel and Chickpeas Provençal 65

    Cabbage Stew 66

    Kimchi Stew 67

    African Peanut Lentil Soup 68

    Spicy Bean Stew 70

    Eggplant, Onion and Tomato Stew 71

    White Bean Stew 72

    Brussel Sprouts Stew 73

    Vegetarian Gumbo 74

    Black Bean and Quinoa Stew 76

    Root Vegetable Stew 77

    Portobello Mushroom Stew 78

Chapter 4.   Beans and Grains **79**

    Garlic and White Bean Soup 79

    Coconut Curry Lentils 80

    Tomato, Kale, and White Bean Skillet 81

    Chard Wraps With Millet 82

    Quinoa Meatballs 83

    Rice Stuffed Jalapeños 84

    Pineapple Fried Rice 85

    Lentil and Wild Rice Soup 86

    Black Bean Meatball Salad 87

    Black Beans and Cauliflower Rice 89

Black Bean Stuffed Sweet Potatoes 90

Black Bean and Quinoa Salad 91

Chickpea Fajitas 92

Coconut Chickpea Curry 94

Mediterranean Chickpea Casserole 95

Zoodles with White Beans..97

Sweet Potato and White Bean Skillet 98

Chapter 5.   Salads **99**

Cauliflower & Apple Salad 99

Corn & Black Bean Salad...100

Spinach & Orange Salad...101

Red Pepper & Broccoli Salad 102

Lentil Potato Salad 103

Black Bean & Corn Salad with Avocado 104

Summer Chickpea Salad 105

Edamame Salad 106

Fruity Kale Salad 107

Olive & Fennel Salad 108

Avocado & Radish Salad 109

Zucchini & Lemon Salad 110

Watercress & Blood Orange Salad... 111

Parsley Salad..112

Tomato Eggplant Spinach Salad..113

Cauliflower Radish Salad 115

Celery Salad 116

Chapter 6.   Desserts & Snacks **117**

Lemon Raspberry Fat Bombs 117

Crunchy Chocolate Brownies 118

Peanut Butter Chocolate Cups 119

Strawberry Cheesecake Bites 120

Chickpea Meringues 121

Spinach and Artichoke Dip 122

Malt Glazed Wheat Thins...124

Potato Chips with Thyme 126

Tofu Spring Rolls..127

Sicilian Eggplant Caponata 128

Conclusion **130**

Introduction

A plant-based diet means eating foods that mostly or entirely made from plants, and it actually allows you meet your nutritional needs by consuming foods in which none or close to none of the ingredients come from animals. A plant-based diet also focuses on healthful whole foods, rather than processed foods.

Plant based diet is rich in nutrients, and if you go from a Western diet to a plant based one, you will stop eating animal products and switch to plant based foods you will start getting more fiber, antioxidants, beneficial plant compounds, magnesium, potassium, vitamins A, C and E, and folate which in result will improve your health. But this type of diet should be carefully planned to achieve that desired result.

Plant based diet may lower the risk of cancer and people on vegan diet may have a 15% lower risk of getting cancer or die from it. It can be effective at reducing symptoms of arthritis such as pain, joint swelling and morning stiffness.

Plant based diet can also help with losing weight. Several trusted studies show that this kind of diet is more efficient when compared with other weight loss diets.

There are several benefits of consuming a plant-based diet. Plants provide three different types of nutrients: macro, micro and phytonutrients. They all work differently and, in conjunction, bring positive effects to human health. Macronutrients ensure a good dose of energy and muscle building, while micronutrients participate in active metabolism. Phytonutrients on the other hand play a role in healing.

Since plants offer a balanced mix of all nutrients, it can prevent weight gain. The reduced amount of cholesterol also balances high blood cholesterol levels and consequently controls blood pressure. People suffering from cardiac problems, cancers, high cholesterol, diabetes and obesity are all, therefore, recommended to consume a plant-based, organic diet. According to a meta-analysis of 343 research studies, organic foods consist of 65 percent antioxidants, which can counter the negative effects of cancer and high blood sugar levels in the case of diabetes. While on this diet, every individual can follow a unique diet plan based on their specific health needs. Here is the list of the diseases a plant-based diet can be most effective in treating.

- Heart attack

- Stroke

- Type I diabetes

- Type II diabetes

- High blood pressure

- Obesity

- Cancers

- High cholesterol levels

This diet can be adopted anytime. Even a slight shift toward a more plant-based way of eating can give you noticeable benefits. These benefits are experienced alike by the young and the old, so you have little to lose by giving it a try.

Enjoy the recipes!

Chapter 1. Breakfast Recipes

Vegan Breakfast Sandwich

Preparation time: 15 minutes
Cooking time: 8 minutes
Servings: 3
Ingredients:
1 cup of spinach
6 slices of pickle
14 oz tofu , extra-firm, pressed
2 medium tomatoes , sliced
1/2 teaspoon garlic powder
¼ teaspoon ground black pepper
1/2 teaspoon black salt
1 teaspoon turmeric
1 tablespoon coconut oil
2 tablespoons vegan mayo
3 slices of vegan cheese
6 slices of gluten-free bread, toasted
Directions:
Cut tofu into six slices, and then season its one side with garlic, black pepper, salt, and turmeric.

Take a skillet pan, place it over medium heat, add oil and when hot, add seasoned tofu slices in it, season side down, and cook for 3 minutes until crispy and light brown.

Then flip the tofu slices and continue cooking for 3 minutes until browned and crispy.

When done, transfer tofu slices on a baking sheet, in the form of a set of two slices side by side, then top each set with a cheese slice and broil for 3 minutes until cheese has melted.

Spread mayonnaise on both sides of slices, top with two slices of tofu, cheese on the side, top with spinach, tomatoes, pickles, and then close the sandwich.

Cut the sandwich into half and then serve.

Nutrition:
Calories: 364 Cal
Fat: 12 g
Carbs: 51 g
Protein: 16 g
Fiber: 3 g

Vegan Fried Egg

Preparation time: 5 minutes

Cooking time: 8 minutes

Servings: 4

Ingredients:

1 block of firm tofu, firm, pressed, drained

½ teaspoon ground black pepper

½ teaspoon salt

1 tablespoon vegan butter

1 cup vegan toast dipping sauce

Directions:

Cut tofu into four slices, and then shape them into a rough circle by using a cookie cutter.

Take a frying pan, place it over medium heat, add butter and when it melts, add prepared tofu slices in a single layer and cook for 3 minutes per side until light brown.

Transfer tofu to serving dishes, make a small hole in the middle of tofu by using a small cookie cutter and fill the hole with dipping sauce.

Garnish eggs with black pepper and sauce and then serve.

Nutrition:

Calories: 86 Cal

Fat: 9 g

Carbs: 0.5 g

Protein: 2 g

Fiber: 0 g

Sweet Crepes

Preparation time: 5 minutes

Cooking time: 8 minutes

Servings: 5

Ingredients:

1 cup of water

1 banana

1/2 cup oat flour

1/2 cup brown rice flour

1 teaspoon baking powder

1 tablespoon coconut sugar

1/8 teaspoon salt

Directions:

Take a blender, place all the ingredients in it except for sugar and salt and pulse for 1 minute until smooth.

Take a skillet pan, place it over medium-high heat, grease it with oil and when hot, pour in ¼ cup of batter, spread it as thin as possible, and cook for 2 to 3 minutes per side until golden brown.

Cook remaining crepes in the same manner, then sprinkle with sugar and salt and serve.

Nutrition:

Calories: 160.1 Cal

Fat: 4.3 g

Carbs: 22 g

Protein: 8.3 g

Fiber: 0.6 g

Spinach Artichoke Quiche

Preparation time: 10 minutes

Cooking time: 55 minutes

Servings: 4

Ingredients:

14 oz tofu, soft

14 oz of artichokes, chopped

2 cups spinach

½ of a large onion, peeled, chopped

1 lemon, juiced

1 teaspoon minced garlic

¼ teaspoon salt

¼ teaspoon ground black pepper

1 teaspoon dried basil

½ teaspoon turmeric

1 tablespoon coconut oil

1 teaspoon Dijon mustard

½ cup nutritional yeast

2 large tortillas, cut into half

Directions:

Switch on the oven, then set it to 350 degrees F and let it preheat.

Take a pie plate, grease it with oil, place tortilla to cover the bottom and sides of the plate and bake for 10 to 15 minutes until baked.

Meanwhile, take a large pan, place it over medium heat, add oil and when hot, add onion and cook for 5 minutes.

Then add garlic, cook for 1 minute until fragrant, stir in spinach and cook for 4 minutes until the spinach has wilted, set aside when done.

Place tofu in a food processor, add all the spices, yeast, and lemon juice and pulse for 2 minutes until smooth.

Then add cooked onion mixture and artichokes, blend for 15 to 25 times until combined, and then pour the mixture over crust in the pie plate.

Bake quiche for 45 minutes until done, then cut it into wedges and serve.

Nutrition:

Calories: 100.3 Cal

Fat: 4.7 g

Carbs: 5 g

Protein: 9.3 g

Fiber: 0.7 g

Tofu Scramble

Preparation time: 5 minutes

Cooking time: 18 minutes

Servings: 4

Ingredients:

For The Spice Mix:

1 teaspoon black salt

1/4 teaspoon garlic powder

1 teaspoon red chili powder

1 teaspoon ground cumin

3/4 teaspoons turmeric

2 tablespoons nutritional yeast

For The Tofu Scramble:

2 cups cooked black beans

16 ounces tofu, firm, pressed, drained

1 chopped red pepper

1 1/2 cups sliced button mushrooms

1/2 of white onion, chopped

1 teaspoon minced garlic

1 tablespoon olive oil

Directions:

Take a skillet pan, place it over medium-high heat, add oil and when hot, add onion, pepper, mushrooms, and garlic and cook for 8 minutes until golden.

Meanwhile, prepare the spice mix and for this, place all its ingredients in a bowl and stir until combined.

When vegetables have cooked, add tofu in it, crumble it, then add black beans, sprinkle with prepared spice mix, stir and cook for 8 minutes until hot.

Serve straight away

Nutrition:

Calories: 175 Cal

Fat: 9 g

Carbs: 10 g

Protein: 14 g

Fiber: 3 g

Pumpkin Muffins

Preparation time: 15 minutes

Cooking time: 30 minutes

Servings: 9

Ingredients:

2 Tablespoon mashed ripe banana

1.5 flax eggs

1 teaspoon vanilla extract, unsweetened

1/4 cup maple syrup

1/4 cup olive oil

2/3 cup coconut sugar

3/4 cup pumpkin puree

1 1/4 teaspoon pumpkin pie spice

1/4 teaspoon sea salt

1/2 teaspoon ground cinnamon

2 teaspoon baking soda

1/2 cup water

1/2 cup almond meal

1 cup gluten-free flour blend

3/4 cup rolled oats

For the Crumble:

2 Tablespoon chopped pecans

3 1/2 Tablespoon gluten-free flour blend

3 Tablespoon coconut sugar

1/8 teaspoon cinnamon

1/8 teaspoon pumpkin pie spice

1 1/4 Tablespoon coconut oil

Directions:

Switch on the oven, then set it to 350 degrees F and let it preheat.

Meanwhile, prepare the muffin batter and for this, place the first seven ingredients in a bowl and whisk until combined.

Then whisk in the next five ingredients until mixed and gradually beat in remaining ingredients until incorporated and smooth batter comes together.

Prepare crumble, and for this, place all of its ingredients in a bowl and stir until combined.

Distribute the batter evenly between ten muffin tins lined with muffin liners, top with prepared crumble, and then bake for 30 minutes until muffins are set and the tops are golden brown.

When done, let muffin cool for 5 minutes, then take them out to cool completely and serve.

Nutrition:

Calories: 329 Cal

Fat: 12.7 g

Carbs: 52.6 g

Protein: 4.6 g

Fiber: 5 g

Tomato and Asparagus Quiche

Preparation time: 40 minutes

Cooking time: 35 minutes

Servings: 12

Ingredients:

For the Dough:

2 cups whole wheat flour

1/2 teaspoon salt

3/4 cup vegan margarine

1/3 cup water

For the Filling:

14 oz silken tofu

6 cherry tomatoes, halved

2 green onions, cut into rings

10 sun-dried tomatoes, in oil, chopped

7 oz green asparagus, diced

1 1/2 tablespoons herbs de Provence

1 tablespoon cornstarch

1 teaspoon turmeric

3 tablespoons olive oil

Directions:

Switch on the oven, then set it to 350 degrees F and let it preheat.

Pre the dough and for this, take a bowl, place all the ingredients for it, beat until incorporated, then knead for 5 minutes until smooth and refrigerate the dough for 30 minutes.

Meanwhile, take a skillet pan, place it over medium heat, add 1 tablespoon oil and when hot, add green onion and cook for 2 minutes, set aside until required.

Place a pot half full wit salty water over medium heat, bring it to boil, then add asparagus and boil for 3 minutes until tender, drain and set aside until required.

Take a medium bowl, add tofu along with herbs de Provence, starch, turmeric, and oil, whisk until smooth and then fold in tomatoes, green onion, and asparagus until mixed.

Divide the prepared dough into twelve sections, take a muffin tray, line it twelve cups with baking cups, and then press a dough ball at the bottom of each cup and all the way up.

Fill the cups with prepared tofu mixture, top with tomatoes, and bake for 35 minutes until cooked.

Serve straight away.

Nutrition:

Calories: 206 Cal

Fat: 14 g

Carbs: 16 g

Protein: 4 g

Fiber: 2 g

Simple Vegan Breakfast Hash

Preparation time: 10 minutes

Cooking time: 25 minutes

Servings: 4

Ingredients:

For The Potatoes:

1 large sweet potato, peeled, diced

3 medium potatoes, peeled, diced

1 tablespoon onion powder

2 teaspoons sea salt

1 tablespoon garlic powder

1 teaspoon ground black pepper

1 teaspoon dried thyme

1/4 cup olive oil

For The Skillet Mixture:

1 medium onion, peeled, diced

5 cloves of garlic, peeled, minced

¼ teaspoon of sea salt

¼ teaspoon ground black pepper

1 teaspoon olive oil

Directions:

Switch on the oven, then set it to 450 degrees F and let it preheat.

Meanwhile, take a casserole dish, add all the ingredients for the potatoes, toss until coated, and then cook for 20 minutes until crispy, stirring halfway.

Meanwhile, take a skillet pan, place it over medium heat, add oil and when hot, add onion and garlic, season with salt and black pepper and cook for 5 minutes until browned.

When potatoes have roasted, add garlic and cooked onion mixture, stir until combined, and serve.

Nutrition:

Calories: 212 Cal

Fat: 10 g

Carbs: 28 g

Protein: 3 g

Fiber: 4 g

Chickpeas On Toast

Preparation time: 5 minutes

Cooking time: 15 minutes

Servings: 6

Ingredients:

14-oz cooked chickpeas

1 cup baby spinach

1/2 cup chopped white onion

1 cup crushed tomatoes

½ teaspoon minced garlic

¼ teaspoon ground black pepper

1/2 teaspoon brown sugar

1 teaspoon smoked paprika powder

1/3 teaspoon sea salt

1 tablespoon olive oil

6 slices of gluten-free bread, toasted

Directions:

Take a frying pan, place it over medium heat, add oil and when hot, add onion and cook for 2 minutes.

Then stir in garlic, cook for 30 seconds until fragrant, stir in paprika and continue cooking for 10 seconds.

Add tomatoes, stir, bring the mixture to simmer, season with black pepper, sugar, and salt and then stir in chickpeas.

Sir, in spinach, cook for 2 minutes until leaves have wilted, then remove the pan from heat and taste to adjust seasoning.

Serve cooked chickpeas on toasted bread.

Nutrition:

Calories: 305 Cal

Fat: 7.6 g

Carbs: 45 g

Protein: 13 g

Fiber: 8 g

Blueberry Muffins

Preparation time: 5 minutes

Cooking time: 15 minutes

Servings: 12

Ingredients:

2 cups fresh blueberries

2 cups all-purpose flour

2½ teaspoons baking powder

½ teaspoon salt

¼ teaspoon baking soda

½ cup and 2tablespoon. sugar

zest of 1 lemon

1 teaspoon apple cider vinegar

¼ cup and 2 tablespoons. canola oil

1 cup of soy milk

1 teaspoon vanilla extract, unsweetened

Directions:

Switch on the oven, then set it to 450 degrees F and let it preheat.

Meanwhile, take a small bowl, add vinegar and milk, whisk until combined, and let it stand to curdle.

Take a large bowl, add flour, salt, baking powder, and soda, and stir until mixed.

Whisk in sugar, lemon zest, oil, and vanilla into soy milk mixture, then gradually whisk in flour mixture until incorporated and fold in berries until combined.

Take a twelve cups muffin tray, grease them with oil, distribute the prepared batter in them and bake for 25 minutes until done and the tops are browned.

Let muffins cool for 5 minutes, then cool them completely and serve.

Nutrition:

Calories: 160 Cal

Fat: 5 g

Carbs: 25 g

Protein: 2 g

Fiber: 2 g

Ultimate Breakfast Sandwich

Preparation time: 40 minutes

Cooking time: 10 minutes

Servings: 4

Ingredients:

For the Tofu:

12 ounces tofu, extra-firm, pressed, drain

1/2 teaspoon garlic powder

1 teaspoon liquid smoke

2 tablespoons nutritional yeast

1 teaspoon Sriracha sauce

2 tablespoons soy sauce

2 tablespoons olive oil

2 tablespoons water

For the Vegan Breakfast Sandwich:

1 large tomato, sliced

4 English muffins, halved, toasted

1 avocado, mashed

Directions:

Prepare tofu, and for this, cut tofu into four slices and set aside.

Stir together remaining ingredients of tofu, pour the mixture into a bag, then add tofu pieces, toss until coated and marinate for 30 minutes.

Take a skillet pan, place it over medium-high heat, add tofu slices along with the marinade and cook for 5 minutes per side.

Prepare sandwich and for this, spread mashed avocado on the inner of the muffin, top with a slice of tofu, layer with a tomato slice and then serve.

Nutrition:

Calories: 277 Cal

Fat: 9.1 g

Carbs: 33.1 g

Protein: 16.1 g

Fiber: 3.6 g

Waffles with Fruits

Preparation time: 10 minutes

Cooking time: 20 minutes

Servings: 4

Ingredients:

1 1/4 cup all-purpose flour

2 teaspoon baking powder

3 tablespoon sugar

1/4 teaspoon salt

2 teaspoon vanilla extract, unsweetened

2 tablespoon coconut oil

1 1/4 cup soy milk

Sliced fruits, for topping

Vegan whipping cream, for topping

Directions:

Switch on the waffle maker and let it preheat.

Meanwhile, place flour in a bowl, stir in salt, baking powder, and sugar and whisk in whisk in remaining ingredients, except for topping, until incorporated.

Ladle the batter into the waffle maker and cook until firm and brown.

When done, top waffles with fruits and whipped cream and serve.

Nutrition:

Calories: 277 Cal

Fat: 8.3 g

Carbs: 42.5 g

Protein: 6.2 g

Fiber: 1.5 g

Chickpea Omelet

Preparation time: 5 minutes

Cooking time: 10 minutes

Servings: 1

Ingredients:

3 Tablespoon chickpea flour

1 small white onion, peeled, diced

½ teaspoon black salt

2 tablespoons chopped the dill

2 tablespoons chopped basil

1/8 teaspoon ground black pepper

2 Tablespoon olive oil

8 Tablespoon water

Directions:

Take a bowl, add flour in it along with salt and black pepper, stir until mixed, and then whisk in water until creamy.

Take a skillet pan, place it over medium heat, add 1 tablespoon oil and when hot, add onion and cook for 4 minutes until cooked.

Add onion to omelet mixture and then stir until combined.

Add remaining oil into the pan, pour in prepared batter, spread evenly, and cook for 3 minutes per side until cooked.

Serve omelet with bread.

Nutrition:

Calories: 150 Cal

Fat: 2 g

Carbs: 24.4 g

Protein: 10.2 g

Fiber: 5.8 g

Scrambled Tofu Breakfast Burrito

Preparation time: 15 minutes

Cooking time: 20 minutes

Servings: 4

Ingredients:

For the Tofu:

12-ounce tofu, extra-firm, pressed

1/4 cup minced parsley

1 ½ teaspoon minced garlic

1 teaspoon nutritional yeast

1/4 teaspoon sea salt

1/2 teaspoon red chili powder

1/2 teaspoon cumin

1 teaspoon olive oil

1 Tablespoon hummus

For the Vegetables:

5 baby potatoes, chopped

1 medium red bell pepper, sliced

2 cups chopped kale

1/2 teaspoon ground cumin

1/8 teaspoon sea salt

1/2 teaspoon red chili powder

1 teaspoon oil

The Rest

4 large tortillas

1 medium avocado, chopped

Cilantro as needed

Salsa as needed

Directions:

Switch on the oven, then set it to 400 degrees F and let it preheat.

Take a baking sheet, add potato and bell pepper, drizzle with oil, season with all the spices, toss until coated and bake for 15 minutes until tender and nicely browned.

Then add kale to the potatoes, cook for 5 minutes, and set aside until required.

In the meantime, take a skillet pan, place it over medium heat, add oil and when hot add tofu, crumble it well and cook for 10 minutes until lightly browned.

In the meantime, take a small bowl, add hummus and remaining ingredients for the tofu and stir until combined.

Add hummus mixture into tofu, stir and cook for 3 minutes, set aside until required.

Assemble the burritos and for this, distribute roasted vegetables on the tortilla, top with tofu, avocado, cilantro, and salsa, roll and then serve.

Nutrition:

Calories: 441 Cal

Fat: 19.6 g

Carbs: 53.5 g

Protein: 16.5 g

Fiber: 8 g

Pancake

Preparation time: 10 minutes

Cooking time: 18 minutes

Servings: 4

Ingredients:

Dry Ingredients:

1 cup buckwheat flour

1/8 teaspoon salt

½ teaspoon gluten-free baking powder

½ teaspoon baking soda

Wet Ingredients:

1 tablespoon almond butter

2 tablespoon maple syrup

1 tablespoon lime juice

1 cup coconut milk, unsweetened

Directions:

Take a medium bowl, add all the dry ingredients and stir until mixed.

Take another bowl, place all the wet ingredients, whisk until combined, and then gradually whisk in dry ingredients mixture until smooth and incorporated.

Take a frying pan, place it over medium heat, add 2 teaspoons oil and when hot, drop in batter and cook for 3 minutes per side until cooked and lightly browned.

Serve pancakes and fruits and maple syrup.

Nutrition:

Calories: 148 Cal

Fat: 8.2 g

Carbs: 15 g

Protein: 4.6 g

Fiber: 1.7 g.

Chapter 2. Lunch Recipes

Cashew Siam Salad

Preparation time: 10 minutes

Cooking time: 3 minutes

Servings: 4

Ingredients:

Salad:

4 cups baby spinach, rinsed, drained

½ cup pickled red cabbage

Dressing:

1-inch piece ginger, finely chopped

1 tsp. chili garlic paste

1 tbsp. soy sauce

½ tbsp. rice vinegar

1 tbsp. sesame oil

3 tbsp. avocado oil

Toppings:

½ cup raw cashews, unsalted

¼ cup fresh cilantro, chopped

Directions:

Put the spinach and red cabbage in a large bowl. Toss to combine and set the salad aside.

Toast the cashews in a frying pan over medium-high heat, stirring occasionally until the cashews are golden brown. This should take about 3 minutes. Turn off the heat and set the frying pan aside.

Mix all the dressing ingredients in a medium-sized bowl and use a spoon to mix them into a smooth dressing.

Pour the dressing over the spinach salad and top with the toasted cashews.

Toss the salad to combine all ingredients and transfer the large bowl to the fridge. Allow the salad to chill for up to one hour – doing so will guarantee a better flavor. Alternatively, the salad can be served right away, topped with the optional cilantro. Enjoy!

Nutritional Value Per Serving:

Calories 236

Carbohydrates 6.1 g

Fats 21.6 g

Protein 4.2 g

Avocado and Cauliflower Hummus

Preparation time: 5 minutes

Cooking time: 25 minutes

Servings: 2

Ingredients:

1 medium cauliflower, stem removed and chopped

1 large Hass avocado, peeled, pitted, and chopped

¼ cup extra virgin olive oil

2 garlic cloves

½ tbsp. lemon juice

½ tsp. onion powder

Sea salt and ground black pepper to taste

2 large carrots

¼ cup fresh cilantro, chopped

Directions:

Preheat the oven to 450°F, and line a baking tray with aluminum foil.

Put the chopped cauliflower on the baking tray and drizzle with 2 tablespoons of olive oil.

Roast the chopped cauliflower in the oven for 20-25 minutes, until lightly brown.

Remove the tray from the oven and allow the cauliflower to cool down.

Add all the ingredients—except the carrots and optional fresh cilantro—to a food processor or blender, and blend the ingredients into a smooth hummus.

Transfer the hummus to a medium-sized bowl, cover, and put it in the fridge for at least 30 minutes.

Take the hummus out of the fridge and, if desired, top it with the optional chopped cilantro and more salt and pepper to taste; serve with the carrot fries, and enjoy!

Nutritional Value Per Serving:

Calories 416

Carbohydrates 8.4 g

Fats 40.3 g

Protein 3.3 g

Raw Zoodles with Avocado 'N Nuts

Preparation time: 10 minutes

Servings: 2

Ingredients:

1 medium zucchini

1½ cups basil

1/3 cup water

5 tbsp. pine nuts

2 tbsp. lemon juice

1 medium avocado, peeled, pitted, sliced

Optional: 2 tbsp. olive oil

6 yellow cherry tomatoes, halved

Optional: 6 red cherry tomatoes, halved

Sea salt and black pepper to taste

Directions:

Add the basil, water, nuts, lemon juice, avocado slices, optional olive oil (if desired), salt, and pepper to a blender.

Blend the ingredients into a smooth mixture. Add more salt and pepper to taste and blend again.

Divide the sauce and the zucchini noodles between two medium-sized bowls for serving, and combine in each.

Top the mixtures with the halved yellow cherry tomatoes, and the optional red cherry tomatoes (if desired); serve and enjoy!

Nutritional Value Per Serving:

Calories 317

Carbohydrates 7.4 g

Fats 28.1 g

Protein 7.2 g

Cauliflower Sushi

Preparation time: 30 minutes

Servings: 4

Ingredients:

Sushi Base:

6 cups cauliflower florets

½ cup vegan cheese

1 medium spring onion, diced

4 nori sheets

Sea salt and pepper to taste

1 tbsp. rice vinegar or sushi vinegar

1 medium garlic clove, minced

Filling:

1 medium Hass avocado, peeled, sliced

½ medium cucumber, skinned, sliced

4 asparagus spears

A handful of enoki mushrooms

Directions:

Put the cauliflower florets in a food processor or blender. Pulse the florets into a rice-like substance. When using readymade cauliflower rice, add this to the blender.

Add the vegan cheese, spring onions, and vinegar to the food processor or blender. Top these ingredients with salt and pepper to taste, and pulse everything into a chunky mixture. Make sure not to turn the ingredients into a puree by pulsing too long.

Taste and add more vinegar, salt, or pepper to taste. Add the optional minced garlic clove to the blender and pulse again for a few seconds.

Lay out the nori sheets and spread the cauliflower rice mixture out evenly between the sheets. Make sure to leave at least 2 inches of the top and bottom edges empty.

Place one or more combinations of multiple filling ingredients along the center of the spread out rice mixture. Experiment with different ingredients per nori sheet for the best flavor.

Roll up each nori sheet tightly. (Using a sushi mat will make this easier.)

Either serve the sushi as a nori roll, or, slice each roll up into sushi pieces.

Serve right away with a small amount of wasabi, pickled ginger, and soy sauce!

Nutritional Value Per Serving:

Calories 189

Carbohydrates 7.6 g

Fats 14.4 g

Protein 6.1 g

Spinach and Mashed Tofu Salad

Preparation time: 20 minutes

Servings: 4

Ingredients:

2 8-oz. blocks firm tofu, drained

4 cups baby spinach leaves

4 tbsp. cashew butter

1½ tbsp. soy sauce

1-inch piece ginger, finely chopped

1 tsp. red miso paste

2 tbsp. sesame seeds

1 tsp. organic orange zest

1 tsp. nori flakes

2 tbsp. water

Directions:

Use paper towels to absorb any excess water left in the tofu before crumbling both blocks into small pieces.

In a large bowl, combine the mashed tofu with the spinach leaves.

Mix the remaining ingredients in another small bowl and, if desired, add the optional water for a more smooth dressing.

Pour this dressing over the mashed tofu and spinach leaves.

Transfer the bowl to the fridge and allow the salad to chill for up to one hour. Doing so will guarantee a better flavor. Or, the salad can be served right away. Enjoy!

Nutritional Value Per Serving:

Calories 166

Carbohydrates 5.5 g

Fats 10.7 g

Protein 11.3 g

Cucumber Edamame Salad

Preparation time: 5 minutes

Cooking time: 8 minutes

Servings: 2

Ingredients:

3 tbsp. avocado oil

1 cup cucumber, sliced into thin rounds

½ cup fresh sugar snap peas, sliced or whole

½ cup fresh edamame

¼ cup radish, sliced

1 large Hass avocado, peeled, pitted, sliced

1 nori sheet, crumbled

2 tsp. roasted sesame seeds

1 tsp. salt

Directions:

Bring a medium-sized pot filled halfway with water to a boil over medium-high heat.

Add the sugar snaps and cook them for about 2 minutes.

Take the pot off the heat, drain the excess water, transfer the sugar snaps to a medium-sized bowl and set aside for now.

Fill the pot with water again, add the teaspoon of salt and bring to a boil over medium-high heat.

Add the edamame to the pot and let them cook for about 6 minutes.

Take the pot off the heat, drain the excess water, transfer the soybeans to the bowl with sugar snaps and let them cool down for about 5 minutes.

Combine all ingredients, except the nori crumbs and roasted sesame seeds, in a medium-sized bowl.

Carefully stir, using a spoon, until all ingredients are evenly coated in oil.

Top the salad with the nori crumbs and roasted sesame seeds.

Transfer the bowl to the fridge and allow the salad to cool for at least 30 minutes.

Serve chilled and enjoy!

Nutritional Value Per Serving:

Calories 409

Carbohydrates 7.1 g

Fats 38.25 g

Protein 7.6 g

Artichoke White Bean Sandwich Spread

Preparation time: 10 minutes

Servings: 2

Ingredients:

½ cup raw cashews, chopped

Water

1 clove garlic, cut into half

1 tablespoon lemon zest

1 teaspoon fresh rosemary, chopped

¼ teaspoon salt

¼ teaspoon pepper

6 tablespoons almond, soy or coconut milk

1 15.5-ounce can cannellini beans, rinsed and drained well

3 to 4 canned artichoke hearts, chopped

¼ cup hulled sunflower seeds

Green onions, chopped, for garnish

Directions:

Soak the raw cashews for 15 minutes in enough water to cover them. Drain and dab with a paper towel to make them as dry as possible.

Transfer the cashews to a blender and add the garlic, lemon zest, rosemary, salt and pepper. Pulse to break everything up and then add the milk, one tablespoon at a time, until the mixture is smooth and creamy.

Mash the beans in a bowl with a fork. Add the artichoke hearts and sunflower seeds. Toss to mix.

Pour the cashew mixture on top and season with more salt and pepper if desired. Mix the ingredients well and spread on whole-wheat bread, crackers, or a wrap.

Nutritional Value Per Serving:

Calories 110

Carbohydrates 14 g

Fats 4 g

Protein 6 g

Buffalo Chickpea Wraps

Preparation time: 20 minutes

Cooking time: 5 minutes

Servings: 4

Ingredients:

¼ cup plus 2 tablespoons hummus

2 tablespoons lemon juice

1½ tablespoons maple syrup

1 to 2 tablespoons hot water

1 head Romaine lettuce, chopped

1 15-ounce can chickpeas, drained, rinsed and patted dry

4 tablespoons hot sauce, divided

1 tablespoon olive or coconut oil

¼ teaspoon garlic powder

1 pinch sea salt

4 wheat tortillas

¼ cup cherry tomatoes, diced

¼ cup red onion, diced

¼ of a ripe avocado, thinly sliced

Directions:

Mix the hummus with the lemon juice and maple syrup in a large bowl. Use a whisk and add the hot water, a little at a time until it is thick but spreadable.

Add the Romaine lettuce and toss to coat. Set aside.

Pour the prepared chickpeas into another bowl. Add three tablespoons of the hot sauce, the olive oil, garlic powder and salt; toss to coat.

Heat a metal skillet (cast iron works the best) over medium heat and add the chickpea mixture. Sauté for three to five minutes and mash gently with a spoon.

Once the chickpea mixture is slightly dried out, remove from the heat and add the rest of the hot sauce. Stir it in well and set aside.

Lay the tortillas on a clean, flat surface and spread a quarter cup of the buffalo chickpeas on top. Top with tomatoes, onion and avocado (optional) and wrap.

Nutritional Value Per Serving:

Calories 254

Carbohydrates 39.4 g

Fats 6.7 g

Protein 9.1 g

Coconut Veggie Wraps

Preparation time: 5 minutes

Servings: 5

Ingredients:

1½ cups shredded carrots

1 red bell pepper, seeded, thinly sliced

2½ cups kale

1 ripe avocado, thinly sliced

1 cup fresh cilantro, chopped

5 coconut wraps

2/3 cups hummus

6½ cups green curry paste

Directions:

Slice, chop and shred all the vegetables.

Lay a coconut wrap on a clean flat surface and spread two tablespoons of the hummus and one tablespoon of the green curry paste on top of the end closest to you.

Place some carrots, bell pepper, kale and cilantro on the wrap and start rolling it up, starting from the edge closest to you. Roll tightly and fold in the ends.

Place the wrap, seam down, on a plate to serve.

Nutritional Value Per Serving:

Calories 236

Carbohydrates 23.6 g

Fats 14.3 g

Protein 5.5 g

Cucumber Avocado Sandwich

Preparation time: 15 minutes

Servings: 2

Ingredients:

½ of a large cucumber, peeled, sliced

¼ teaspoon salt

4 slices whole-wheat bread

4 ounces goat cheese with or without herbs, at room temperature

2 Romaine lettuce leaves

1 large avocado, peeled, pitted, sliced

2 pinches lemon pepper

1 squeeze of lemon juice

½ cup alfalfa sprouts

Directions:

Peel and slice the cucumber thinly. Lay the slices on a plate and sprinkle them with a quarter to a half teaspoon of salt. Let this set for 10 minutes or until water appears on the plate.

Place the cucumber slices in a colander and rinse with cold water. Let these drain, then place them on a dry plate and pat dry with a paper towel.

Spread all slices with goat cheese and place lettuce leaves on the two bottom pieces of bread.

Layer the cucumber slices and avocado atop the bread.

Sprinkle one pinch of lemon pepper over each sandwich and drizzle a little lemon juice over the top.

Top with the alfalfa sprouts and place another piece of bread, goat cheese down, on top.

Nutritional Value Per Serving:

Calories 246

Carbohydrates 20 g

Fats 12 g

Protein 9 g

Lentil Sandwich Spread

Preparation time: 15 minutes

Cooking time: 20 minutes

Servings: 3

Ingredients:

1 tablespoon water or oil

1 small onion, chopped

2 cloves garlic, minced

1 cup dry lentils

2 cups vegetable stock

1 tablespoon apple cider vinegar

2 tablespoons tomato paste

3 sun-dried tomatoes

2 tablespoons maple

1 teaspoon dried oregano

½ teaspoon ground cumin

1 teaspoon coriander

1 teaspoon turmeric

½ lemon, juiced

1 tablespoon fresh parsley, chopped

Directions:

Warm a Dutch oven over medium heat and add the water or oil.

Immediately add the onions and sauté for two to three minutes or until softened. Add more water if this starts to stick to the pan.

Add the garlic and sauté for one minute.

Add the lentils, vegetable stock and vinegar; bring to a boil. Turn down to a simmer and cook for 15 minutes or until the lentils are soft and the liquid is almost completely absorbed.

Ladle the lentils into a food processor and add the tomato paste, sun-dried tomatoes and syrup; process until smooth.

Add the oregano, cumin, coriander, turmeric and lemon; processes until thoroughly mixed.

Remove the spread to a bowl and apply it to bread, toast, a wrap, or pita. Sprinkle With toppings as desired.

Nutritional Value Per Serving:

Calories 360

Carbohydrates 60.7 g

Fats 5.4 g

Protein 17.5 g

Mediterranean Tortilla Pinwheels

Preparation time: 5 minutes

Cooking time: 1 minute

Servings: 16

Ingredients:

½ cup water

4 tablespoons white vinegar

3 tablespoons lemon juice

3 tablespoons tahini paste

1 clove garlic, minced

Salt and pepper to taste

Canned artichokes, drained, thinly sliced

Cherry tomatoes, thinly sliced

Olives, thinly sliced

Lettuce or baby spinach

Tortillas

Directions:

In a bowl, combine the water, vinegar, lemon juice and Tahini paste; whisk together until smooth.

Add the garlic, salt and pepper to taste; whisk to combine. Set the bowl aside.

Lay a tortilla on a flat surface and spread with one tablespoon of the sauce.

Lay some lettuce or spinach slices on top, then scatter some artichoke, tomato and olive slices on top.

Tightly roll the tortilla and fold in the sides. Cut the ends off and then slice into four or five pinwheels.

Nutritional Value Per Serving:

Calories 322

Carbohydrates 5 g

Fats 4 g

Protein 30 g

Rice and Bean Burritos

Preparation time: 10 minutes

Cooking time: 15 minutes

Servings: 8

Ingredients:

2 16-ounce cans fat-free refried beans

6 tortillas

2 cups cooked rice

½ cup salsa

1 tablespoon olive oil

1 bunch green onions, chopped

2 bell peppers, finely chopped

Guacamole

Directions:

Preheat the oven to 375°F.

Dump the refried beans into a saucepan and place over medium heat to warm.

Heat the tortillas and lay them out on a flat surface.

Spoon the beans in a long mound that runs across the tortilla, just a little off from center.

Spoon some rice and salsa over the beans; add the green pepper and onions to taste, along with any other finely chopped vegetables you like.

Fold over the shortest edge of the plain tortilla and roll it up, folding in the sides as you go.

Place each burrito, seam side down, on a nonstick-sprayed baking sheet.

Brush with olive oil and bake for 15 minutes.

Serve with guacamole.

Nutritional Value Per Serving:

Calories 290

Carbohydrates 49 g

Fats 6 g

Protein 9 g

Ricotta Basil Pinwheels

Prep: 10 minutes

Serves 4

Ingredients:

½ cup unsalted cashews

Water

7 ounces firm tofu, cut into pieces

¼ cup almond milk

1 teaspoon white wine vinegar

1 clove garlic, smashed

20 to 25 fresh basil leaves

Salt and pepper to taste

8 tortillas

7 ounces fresh spinach

½ cup black olives, sliced

2 to 3 tomatoes, cut into small pieces

Directions:

Soak the cashews for 30 minutes in enough water to cover them. Drain them well and pat them dry with paper towels.

Place the cashews in a blender along with the tofu, almond milk, vinegar, garlic, basil leaves, salt and pepper to taste. Blend until smooth and creamy.

Spread the resulting mixture on the eight tortillas, dividing it equally.

Top with spinach leaves, olives and tomatoes.

Tightly roll each loaded tortilla.

Cut off the ends with a sharp knife and slice into four or five pinwheels.

Delicious Sloppy Joes With No Meat

Preparation time: 6 minutes

Cooking time: 5 minutes

Servings: 4

Ingredients:

5 tablespoons vegetable stock

2 stalks celery, diced

1 small onion, diced

1 small red bell pepper, diced

1 teaspoon garlic powder

1 teaspoon chili powder

1 teaspoon ground cumin

1 teaspoon salt

1 cup cooked bulgur wheat

1 cup red lentils

1 15-ounce can tomato sauce

4 tablespoons tomato paste

3½ cups water

2 teaspoons balsamic vinegar

1 tablespoon Hoisin sauce

Directions:

In a Dutch oven, heat up the vegetable stock and add the celery, onion and bell pepper. Sauté until vegetables are soft, about five minutes.

Add the garlic powder, chili powder, cumin and salt and mix in.

Add the bulgur wheat, lentils, tomato sauce, tomato paste, water, vinegar and Hoisin sauce. Stir and bring to a boil.

Turn the heat down to a simmer and cook uncovered for 30 minutes. Stir occasionally to prevent sticking and scorching.

Taste to see if the lentils are tender.

When the lentils are done, serve on buns.

Nutritional Value Per Serving:

Calories 451

Fats 10 g

Carbohydrates 61 g

Protein 27 g

Spicy Hummus and Apple Wrap

Preparation time: 10 minutes

Servings: 1

Ingredients:

3 to 4 tablespoons hummus

2 tablespoons mild salsa

½ cup broccoli slaw

½ teaspoon fresh lemon juice

2 teaspoons plain yogurt

salt and pepper to taste

1 tortilla

Lettuce leaves

½ Granny Smith or another tart apple, cored and thinly sliced

Directions:

In a small bowl, mix the hummus with the salsa. Set the bowl aside.

In a large bowl, mix the broccoli slaw, lemon juice and yogurt. Season with the salt and pepper.

Lay the tortilla on a flat surface and spread on the hummus mixture.

Lay down some lettuce leaves on top of the hummus.

On the upper half of the tortilla, place a pile of the broccoli slaw mixture and cover with the apples.

Fold and wrap.

Nutritional Value Per Serving:

Calories 121

Carbohydrates 27 g

Fats 2 g

Protein 4 g

Sun-dried Tomato Spread

Preparation time: 20 minutes

Servings: 16

Ingredients:

1 cup sun-dried tomatoes

1 cup raw cashews

Water for soaking tomatoes and cashews

½ cup water

1 clove garlic, minced

1 green onion, chopped

5 large basil leaves

½ teaspoon lemon juice

¼ teaspoon salt

1 dash pepper

Hulled sunflower seeds

Directions:

Soak tomatoes and cashews for 30 minutes in separate bowls, with enough water to cover them. Drain and pat dry.

Put the tomatoes and cashews in a food processor and puree them, drizzling the water in as it purees to make a smooth, creamy paste.

Add the garlic, onion, basil leaves, lemon juice, salt and pepper and mix thoroughly.

Scrape into a bowl, cover and refrigerate overnight.

Spread on bread or toast and sprinkle with sunflower seeds for a little added crunch.

Nutritional Value Per Serving:

Calories 60

Carbohydrates 5.6 g

Fats 4.2 g

Protein 1.2 g

Sweet Potato Sandwich Spread

Preparation time: 10 minutes

Servings: 4

Ingredients:

1 large sweet potato baked, peeled

1 teaspoon cumin

1 teaspoon chili powder

1 teaspoon garlic powder

Salt and pepper to taste

2 slices whole-wheat bread

1 to 2 tablespoons pinto beans, drained

Lettuce

Directions:

Bake and peel the sweet potato and mash it in a bowl. If it is too thick, add a little almond or coconut milk.

Mix in the cumin, chili powder, garlic powder, salt and pepper.

Spread the mixture on a slice of bread and spoon some beans on top.

Top with lettuce leaves and the other slice of bread.

Nutritional Value Per Serving:

Calories 253

Carbohydrates 49 g

Fats 6 g

Protein 8 g

Zucchini Sandwich with Balsamic Dressing

Preparation time: 5 minutes

Cooking time: 2 minutes

Servings: 2

Ingredients:

2 small zucchinis

1 tablespoon olive oil

4 cloves garlic, thinly sliced

1 tablespoon balsamic vinegar

1 large roasted red pepper, chopped

1 cup cannellini beans, rinsed, drained

2 whole-wheat sandwich rolls

6 to 8 basil leaves

½ teaspoon pepper

Directions:

Add the oil to a hot skillet and sauté the garlic for one or two minutes or until it just starts to brown.

Add the zucchini strips and sauté in batches (don't overcrowd) and lay out on a plate until they are all finished.

Reduce heat to medium and place all the zucchini strips back in the pan.

Add the vinegar and sauté for about a minute.

In the blender, process the red pepper and beans until smooth.

Toast the buns and spoon onto the bottom halves the bean and pepper mixture.

Lay basil leaves on top and then the zucchini.

Grind some pepper on top and close the sandwich with the top of the bun.

Nutritional Value Per Serving:

Calories 274

Carbohydrates 50.1 g

Fats 2.5 g

Protein 16 g

Chapter 3. Soup Recipes

Butternut Squash and Coconut Milk Soup

Preparation time: 10 minutes

Cooking time: 35 minutes

Servings: 6

Ingredients:

1 cup diced parsnips

2 cups diced sweet potato

1 large sweet onion, peeled, diced

1 ½ cups diced carrots

4 cups diced butternut squash

2 teaspoons minced garlic

1/4 teaspoon ground ginger

¼ teaspoon ground black pepper

½ teaspoon of sea salt

1/4 teaspoon ground allspice

1 teaspoon poultry seasoning

1 teaspoon pumpkin pie spice

1/4 teaspoon ground cinnamon

32 ounces vegetable stock

14 ounces coconut milk, unsweetened

Directions:

Take a large Dutch oven, place it over medium heat, add onions, drizzle with 2 tablespoons water and cook for 5 minutes until softened, drizzling with more 2 tablespoons at a time if required.

Then stir in garlic, cook for another minute, switch heat to the high level, add remaining ingredients, reserving milk, salt, and black pepper, and bring the soup to boil.

Then switch heat to medium-low level and simmer for 20 minutes until vegetables are tender.

When done, puree soup by using an immersion blender, then stir in coconut milk, season with salt and black pepper and cook for 3 minutes until warm.

Serve straight away.

Nutrition Value:

Calories: 188.4 Cal

Fat: 7.7 g

Carbs: 29.3 g

Protein: 3.7 g

Fiber: 8.2 g

Broccoli Cheese Soup

Preparation time: 10 minutes

Cooking time: 15 minutes

Servings: 4

Ingredients:

1 medium potato, peeled, diced

2 ribs celery, diced

1 medium white onion, peeled, diced

2 medium yellow summer squash, diced

1 medium carrot, peeled, diced

6 cups chopped broccoli florets

1 teaspoon minced garlic

1 bay leaf

1/3 teaspoon ground black pepper

¼ cup nutritional yeast

1 tablespoon lemon juice

2 tablespoons apple cider vinegar

½ cup cashews

3 cups of water

Directions:

Take a large pot, place it over medium-high heat, add all the vegetables in it, except for florets, add bay leaf, pour in water and bring the mixture to boil.

Then switch heat to medium-low and simmer for 10 minutes until vegetables are tender.

Meanwhile, place broccoli florets in another pot, place it over medium-low heat and cook for 4 minutes or more until broccoli has steamed.

When done, remove broccoli from the pot, reserve 1 cup of its liquid, and set aside until required.

When vegetables have cooked, remove the bay leaf, add remaining ingredients in it, reserving broccoli and its liquid, and then puree the soup by using an immersion blender until smooth.

Then add steamed broccoli along with its liquid, stir well and serve straight away.

Nutrition Value:

Calories: 223.5 Cal

Fat: 12 g

Carbs: 19 g

Protein: 10.6 g

Fiber: 1.7 g

Potato and Kale Soup

Preparation time: 5 minutes

Cooking time: 15 minutes

Servings: 2

Ingredients:

1 small white onion, peeled, chopped

2 ½ cups cubed potatoes

2 cups leek, cut into rings

1/2 cup chopped carrots

1/2 cup chopped celery

½ teaspoon minced garlic

2/3 teaspoon salt

1/3 teaspoon ground black pepper

1 tablespoon olive oil

3 1/2 cups vegetable broth

1 cup kale, cut into stripes

Croutons, for serving

Directions:

Take a large pot, place it over medium heat, add oil and when hot, add onion and cook for 2 minutes until sauté.

Stir in garlic, cook for another minute, then add all the vegetables and continue cooking for 3 minutes.

Pour in broth, cook for 15 minutes, then add kale and cook for 2 minutes until tender.

Season soup with salt and black pepper, puree by using an immersion blender until smooth, then top with croutons and serve.

Nutrition Value:

Calories: 337 Cal

Fat: 7 g

Carbs: 62 g

Protein: 10 g

Fiber: 8 g

Vegan Pho

Preparation time: 5 minutes

Cooking time: 15 minutes

Servings: 6

Ingredients:

1 package of wide rice noodles, cooked

1 medium white onion, peeled, quartered

2 teaspoons minced garlic

1 inch of ginger, sliced into coins

8 cups vegetable broth

3 whole cloves

2 tablespoons soy sauce

3 whole star anise

1 cinnamon stick

3 cups of water

For Toppings:

Basil as needed for topping

Chopped green onions as needed for topping

Ming beans as needed for topping

Hot sauce as needed for topping

Lime wedges for serving

Directions:

Take a large pot, place it over medium-high heat, add all the ingredients for soup in it, except for soy sauce and broth, and bring it to boil.

Then switch heat to medium-low level, simmer the soup for 30 minutes and then stir in soy sauce.

When done, distribute cooked noodles into bowls, top with soup, then top with toppings and serve.

Nutrition Value:

Calories: 31 Cal

Fat: 0 g

Carbs: 7 g

Protein: 0 g

Fiber: 2 g

Roasted Cauliflower Soup

Preparation time: 10 minutes

Cooking time: 60 minutes

Servings: 4

Ingredients:

1 medium head of cauliflower, cut into florets

1 small white onion, peeled, diced

1 medium carrot, peeled, diced

1 stalk of celery, diced

1 head of garlic, top off

2/3 teaspoon salt

1/3 teaspoon ground black pepper

1 teaspoon smoked paprika

2 tablespoons nutritional yeast

1 teaspoon hot smoked paprika

4 tablespoons olive oil

12 ounces coconut milk, unsweetened

4 cups vegetable broth

½ cup chopped parsley

Directions:

Switch on the oven, then set it to 400 degrees F and let it preheat.

Place top off garlic on a piece of foil, drizzle with 1 tablespoon oil, and then wrap.

Place cauliflower florets in a bowl, drizzle with 2 tablespoons oil, season with salt and black pepper, and toss until well coated.

Take a baking sheet, spread cauliflower florets in it in a single layer, add wrapped garlic and bake for 30 minutes until roasted.

Then place a large pot over medium-high heat, add remaining oil and when hot, add onions and cook for 3 minutes.

Then add celery and carrot, continue cooking for 3 minutes, season with salt and paprika, pour in broth, and bring it to a boil.

Add roasted garlic and florets, bring the mixture to boil, then switch heat to medium-low level and simmer for 15 minutes.

Puree the soup by using an immersion blender, stir in milk and yeast until mixed and simmer for 3 minutes until hot.

Garnish soup with parsley and then serve.

Nutrition Value:

Calories: 102.2 Cal

Fat: 6.3 g

Carbs: 11 g

Protein: 2.7 g

Fiber: 4.6 g

Curried Apple and Sweet Potato Soup

Preparation time: 10 minutes

Cooking time: 38 minutes

Servings: 6

Ingredients:

2 cups diced sweet apples

1/2 of medium white onion, peeled chopped

4 cups diced sweet potatoes

1 teaspoon minced garlic

1 tablespoon grated ginger

1/4 teaspoon nutmeg

1 teaspoon curry powder

2/3 teaspoon salt

1/3 teaspoon ground black pepper

1/2 teaspoon cinnamon

1 tablespoon olive oil

2 cups apple cider

1 cup vegetable stock

1 cup coconut milk, unsweetened

For Garnish:

1/2 cup baked apple chips

1/4 cup toasted pumpkin seeds

1/4 cup coconut milk, unsweetened

Directions:

Take a large pot, place it over medium-high heat and when hot, add oil and onion and cook 5 minutes until translucent.

Add garlic and ginger, stir in all the spices, then add sweet potatoes and cook for 4 minutes until sauté.

Switch heat to medium-low level, add apples, pour in milk, stock, and cider coconut and simmer 25 minutes until vegetables are softened.

Puree the soup by using an immersion blender, season with salt and black pepper, and distribute into bowls.

Top with garnishing and then serve.

Nutrition Value:

Calories: 170 Cal

Fat: 8.4 g

Carbs: 22 g

Protein: 3.1 g

Fiber: 5 g

Ramen Noodle Soup

Preparation time: 10 minutes

Cooking time: 20 minutes

Servings: 2

Ingredients:

For The Mushrooms and Tofu:

2 cups sliced shiitake mushrooms

6 ounces tofu, extra-firm, drained, sliced

1 tablespoon olive oil

1 tablespoon soy sauce

For the Noodle Soup:

2 packs of dried ramen noodles

1 medium carrot, peeled, grated

1 inch of ginger, grated

1 teaspoon minced garlic

¾ cup baby spinach leaves

1 tablespoon olive oil

6 cups vegetable broth

For Garnish:

Sesame seeds as needed

Soy sauce as needed

Sriracha sauce as needed

Directions:

Prepare mushrooms and tofu and for this, place tofu pieces in a plastic bag, add soy sauce, seal the bag and turn it upside until tofu is coated.

Take a skillet pan, place it over medium heat, add oil and when hot, add tofu slices and cook for 5 to 10 minutes until crispy and browned on all sides, flipping frequently and when done, set aside until required.

Add mushrooms into the pan, cook for 8 minutes until golden, pour soy sauce from tofu pieces in it, and stir until coated.

Meanwhile, prepare noodle soup and for this, take a soup pot, place it over medium-high heat, add oil and when hot, add garlic and ginger and cook for 1 minute until fragrant.

Then pour in the broth, bring the mixture to boil, add noodles and cook until tender.

Then stir spinach into the noodle soup, remove the pot from heat and distribute evenly between bowls.

Add mushrooms and tofu along with garnishing and then serve.

Nutrition Value:

Calories: 647 Cal

Fat: 12 g

Carbs: 106 g

Protein: 28 g

Fiber: 6 g

Lasagna Soup

Preparation time: 5 minutes

Cooking time: 5 hours and 12 minutes

Servings: 6

Ingredients:

For the Lasagna Soup:

3/4 cup dried brown lentils

1 medium white onion, peeled, diced

3 cups chopped spinach leaves

14 ounces crushed tomatoes

14 ounces diced tomatoes

1 ½ teaspoon minced garlic

1 teaspoon dried basil

1 teaspoon dried oregano

8 lasagna noodles, broken into pieces

4 1/2 cups vegetable broth

For the Vegan Pesto Ricotta:

1/4 pound tofu, extra firm, drained

1 cup cashews, soaked, drained

2/3 teaspoon salt

1/3 teaspoon ground black pepper

4 tablespoons pesto, vegan

1 tablespoon lemon juice

1/4 cup almond milk

Directions:

Prepare the lasagna soup and for this, switch on the slow cooker, add lentils, onion, and garlic in it, stir in basil and oregano, pour in broth, and stir until mixed.

Shut the slow cooker with lid and cook for 2 hours at a high heat setting.

Meanwhile, prepare the pesto ricotta, and for this, place cashews in a blender, add milk and pulse until smooth.

Then tofu, pulse until mixture resembles ricotta cheese, then tip it in a bowl and stir in remaining ingredients until combined, set aside until required.

Then stir in all the tomatoes, continue cooking for 3 hours at high heat setting, add noodles and spinach, stir until mixed and cook for 12 minutes until spinach leaves have wilted.

When done, season the soup with salt and black pepper and then serve with prepared pesto ricotta.

Nutrition Value:

Calories: 450 Cal

Fat: 16.8 g

Carbs: 55.2 g

Protein: 22.6 g

Fiber: 13.2 g

Hot and Sour Soup

Preparation time: 5 minutes

Cooking time: 20 minutes

Servings: 4

Ingredients:

2 tablespoons dried wood ears

3.5 ounces bamboo shoots, sliced into thin strips

1 medium carrot, peeled, sliced into thin strips

5 dried shiitake mushrooms

1 tablespoon grated ginger

1 teaspoon minced garlic

1 teaspoon ground black pepper

1 teaspoon salt

1/4 cup soy sauce

1 teaspoon sugar

1/2 cup rice vinegar

4 cups vegetable stock

1 1/2 cup water, boiling

7.5 ounces tofu, extra-firm, drained

1 tablespoon green onion tops, chopped

¼ cup water, at room temperature

2 tablespoons cornstarch

1 teaspoon sesame oil

Directions:

Take a small bowl, place wood ears in it, then pour in boiling water until covered and let stand for 30 minutes.

Meanwhile, take another bowl, place mushrooms in it, pour in 1 ½ cup water and let the mushrooms stand for 30 minutes.

After 30 minutes, drain the wood ears, rinse well and cut into slices, remove and discard the hard bits.

Similarly, drain the mushrooms, reserving their soaking liquid and slice the mushrooms, removing and discarding their stems.

Take a large pot, place it over medium-high heat, add all the ingredients including reserved mushroom liquid, leave the last five ingredients, stir well and bring the mixture to boil.

Then switch heat to medium level and simmer the soup for 10 minutes until cooked.

Meanwhile, place cornstarch in a bowl, add water at room temperature, and stir well until smooth.

Cut tofu into 1-inch pieces, add into the simmering soup along with cornstarch mixture, and continue to simmer the soup until it reaches to desired thickness.

Drizzle with sesame oil, distribute soup into bowls, garnish with green onions and serve.

Nutrition Value:

Calories: 152 Cal

Fat: 2 g

Carbs: 35 g

Protein: 4 g

Fiber: 8 g

Potato and Corn Chowder

Preparation time: 5 minutes

Cooking time: 16 minutes

Servings: 6

Ingredients:

1 tablespoon olive oil

2 medium carrots, peeled, chopped

2 ribs celery, chopped

1 medium white onion, peeled, chopped

1 ½ teaspoon minced garlic

1/4 cup all-purpose flour

1 teaspoon dried thyme

4 cups chopped white potatoes

2 cups vegetable broth

2 cups almond milk, unsweetened

3 tablespoons nutritional yeast

1 cup frozen corn kernels

1 teaspoon salt

1/4 teaspoon ground black pepper

Directions:

Take a large pot, place it over medium-high heat, add oil and when hot, add onion, carrots, celery, and garlic and cook for 5 minutes until golden brown.

Then sprinkle with flour and thyme, stir until coated, cook for 1 minute until the flour has browned, then add yeast, potatoes, milk, and broth and stir until mixed.

Bring the mixture to simmer, cook for 8 minutes until tender, then add corn and season the soup with salt and black pepper.

Serve straight away.

Nutrition Value:

Calories: 126 Cal

Fat: 3 g

Carbs: 18 g

Protein: 6 g

Fiber: 3 g

Thai Coconut Soup

Preparation time: 10 minutes

Cooking time: 15 minutes

Servings: 12

Ingredients:

2 mangos, peeled, cut into bite-size pieces

1/2 cup green lentils, cooked

2 sweet potatoes, peeled, cubed

1/2 cup quinoa, cooked

1 green bell pepper, cored, cut into strips

½ teaspoon chopped basil

½ teaspoon chopped rosemary

2 tablespoons red curry paste

1/4 cup mixed nut

2 teaspoons orange zest

30 ounces coconut milk, unsweetened

Directions:

Take a large saucepan, place it over medium-high heat, add sweet potatoes, pour in the milk and bring the mixture to boil.

Then switch heat to medium-low level, add remaining ingredients, except for quinoa and lentils, stir and cook for 15 minutes until vegetables have softened.

Then stir in quinoa and lentils, cook for 3 minutes until hot, and then serve.

Nutrition Value:

Calories: 232 Cal

Fat: 19.8 g

Carbs: 10.2 g

Protein: 7.8 g

Fiber: 0.8 g

Spanish Chickpea and Sweet Potato Stew

Preparation time: 5 minutes

Cooking time: 35 minutes

Servings: 4

Ingredients:

14 ounces cooked chickpeas

1 small sweet potato, peeled, cut into ½-inch cubes

1 medium red onion, sliced

3 ounces baby spinach

14 ounces crushed tomatoes

2 teaspoons minced garlic

1 teaspoon salt

1 1/2 teaspoons ground cumin

2 teaspoons harissa paste

2 teaspoons maple syrup

½ teaspoon ground black pepper

2 teaspoons sugar

1 tablespoon olive oil

1/2 cup vegetable stock

2 tablespoons chopped parsley

1 ounce slivered almonds, toasted

Brown rice, cooked, for serving

Directions:

Take a large saucepan, place it over low heat, add oil and when hot, add onion and garlic and cook for 5 minutes.

Then add sweet potatoes, season with cumin, stir in harissa paste and cook for 2 minutes until toasted.

Switch heat to medium-low level, add tomatoes and chickpeas, pour in vegetable stock, stir in maple syrup and sugar and simmer for 25 minutes until potatoes have softened, stirring every 10 minutes.

Then add spinach, cook for 1 minute until its leaves have wilted, and season with salt and black pepper.

When done, distribute cooked rice between bowls, top with stew, garnish with parsley and almonds and serve.

Nutrition Value:

Calories: 348 Cal

Fat: 16.5 g

Carbs: 41.2 g

Protein: 7.2 g

Fiber: 5.3 g

Pomegranate and Walnut Stew

Preparation time: 10 minutes

Cooking time: 55 minutes

Servings: 6

Ingredients:

1 head of cauliflower, cut into florets

1 medium white onion, peeled, diced

1 1/2 cups California walnuts, toasted

1 cup yellow split peas

1 1/2 tablespoons honey

¼ teaspoon salt

½ teaspoon turmeric

½ teaspoon cinnamon

2 tablespoons olive oil, separated

4 cups pomegranate juice

2 tablespoons chopped parsley

2 tablespoons chopped walnuts, for garnishing

Directions:

Take a medium saute pan, place it over medium heat, add walnuts, cook for 5 minutes until toasted and then cool for 5 minutes.

Transfer walnuts to the food processor, pulse for 2 minutes until ground, and set aside until required.

Take a large saute pan, place it over medium heat, add 1 tablespoon oil and when hot, add onion and cook for 5 minutes until softened.

Switch heat to medium-low heat, then add lentils and walnuts, stir in cinnamon, salt, and turmeric, pour in honey and pomegranate, stir until mixed and simmer the mixture for 40 minutes until the sauce has reduced by half and lentils have softened.

Meanwhile, place cauliflower florets in a food processor and then pulse for 2 minutes until mixture resembles rice.

Take a medium to saute pan, place it over medium heat, add remaining oil and when hot, add cauliflower rice, cook for 5 minutes until softened, and then season with salt.

Serve cooked pomegranate and walnut sauce with cooked cauliflower rice and garnish with walnuts and parsley.

Nutrition Value:

Calories: 439 Cal

Fat: 25 g

Carbs: 67 g

Protein: 21 g

Fiber: 3 g

Sweet Potato, Kale and Peanut Stew

Preparation time: 10 minutes

Cooking time: 45 minutes

Servings: 3

Ingredients:

1/4 cup red lentils

2 medium sweet potatoes, peeled, cubed

1 medium white onion, peeled, diced

1 cup kale, chopped

2 tomatoes, diced

1/4 cup chopped green onion

1 teaspoon minced garlic

1 inch of ginger, grated

2 tablespoons toasted peanuts

1/4 teaspoon ground black pepper

1 teaspoon ground cumin

1/2 teaspoon turmeric

1/8 teaspoon cayenne pepper

1 tablespoon peanut butter

1 1/2 cups vegetable broth

2 teaspoons coconut oil

Directions:

Take a medium pot, place it medium heat, add oil and when it melts, add onions and cook for 5 minutes.

Then stir in ginger and garlic, cook for 2 minutes until fragrant, add lentils and potatoes along with all the spices, and stir until mixed.

Stir in tomatoes, pour in the broth, bring the mixture to boil, then switch heat to the low level and simmer for 30 minutes until cooked.

Then stir in peanut butter until incorporated and then puree by using an immersion blender until half-pureed.

Return stew over low heat, stir in kale, cook for 5 minutes until its leaves wilts, and then season with black pepper and salt.

Garnish the stew with peanuts and green onions and then serve.

Nutrition Value:

Calories: 401 Cal

Fat: 6.7 g

Carbs: 77.3 g

Protein: 10.8 g

Fiber: 16 g

Vegetarian Irish Stew

Preparation time: 5 minutes

Cooking time: 38 minutes

Servings: 6

Ingredients:

1 cup textured vegetable protein, chunks

½ cup split red lentils

2 medium onions, peeled, sliced

1 cup sliced parsnip

2 cups sliced mushrooms

1 cup diced celery,

1/4 cup flour

4 cups vegetable stock

1 cup rutabaga

1 bay leaf

½ cup fresh parsley

1 teaspoon sugar

¼ teaspoon ground black pepper

1/4 cup soy sauce

¼ teaspoon thyme

2 teaspoons marmite

¼ teaspoon rosemary

2/3 teaspoon salt

¼ teaspoon marjoram

Directions:

Take a large soup pot, place it over medium heat, add oil and when it gets hot, add onions and cook for 5 minutes until softened.

Then switch heat to the low level, sprinkle with flour, stir well, add remaining ingredients, stir until combined and simmer for 30 minutes until vegetables have cooked.

When done, season the stew with salt and black pepper and then serve.

Nutrition Value:

Calories: 117.4 Cal

Fat: 4 g

Carbs: 22.8 g

Protein: 6.5 g

Fiber: 7.3 g

White Bean and Cabbage Stew

Preparation time: 5 minutes

Cooking time: 8 hours

Servings: 4

Ingredients:

3 cups cooked great northern beans

1.5 pounds potatoes, peeled, cut in large dice

1 large white onion, peeled, chopped

½ head of cabbage, chopped

3 ribs celery, chopped

4 medium carrots, peeled, sliced

14.5 ounces diced tomatoes

1/3 cup pearled barley

1 teaspoon minced garlic

½ teaspoon ground black pepper

1 bay leaf

1 teaspoon dried thyme

½ teaspoon crushed rosemary

1 teaspoon salt

½ teaspoon caraway seeds

1 tablespoon chopped parsley

8 cups vegetable broth

Directions:

Switch on the slow cooker, then add all the ingredients except for salt, parsley, tomatoes, and beans and stir until mixed.

Shut the slow cooker with lid, and cook for 7 hours at low heat setting until cooked.

Then stir in remaining ingredients, stir until combined and continue cooking for 1 hour.

Serve straight away

Nutrition Value:

Calories: 150 Cal

Fat: 0.7 g

Carbs: 27 g

Protein: 7 g

Fiber: 9.4 g

Spinach and Cannellini Bean Stew

Preparation time: 10 minutes

Cooking time: 15 minutes

Servings: 6

Ingredients:

28 ounces cooked cannellini beans

24 ounces tomato passata

17 ounces spinach chopped

¼ teaspoon ground black pepper

2/3 teaspoon salt

1 ¼ teaspoon curry powder

1 cup cashew butter

¼ teaspoon cardamom

2 tablespoons olive oil

1 teaspoon salt

¼ cup cashews

2 tablespoons chopped basil

2 tablespoons chopped parsley

Directions:

Take a large saucepan, place it over medium heat, add 1 tablespoon oil and when hot, add spinach and cook for 3 minutes until fried.

Then stir in butter and tomato passata until well mixed, bring the mixture to a near boil, add beans and season with ¼ teaspoon curry powder, black pepper, and salt.

Take a small saucepan, place it over medium heat, add remaining oil, stir in cashew, stir in salt and curry powder and cook for 4 minutes until roasted, set aside until required.

Transfer cooked stew into a bowl, top with roasted cashews, basil, and parsley, and then serve.

Nutrition Value:

Calories: 242 Cal

Fat: 10.2 g

Carbs: 31 g

Protein: 11 g

Fiber: 8.5 g

Fennel and Chickpeas Provençal

Preparation time: 10 minutes

Cooking time: 50 minutes

Servings: 4

Ingredients:

15 ounces cooked chickpeas

3 fennel bulbs, sliced

1 medium onion, peeled, sliced

15 ounces diced tomatoes

10 black olives, pitted, cured

10 Kalamata olives, pitted

1 ½ teaspoon minced garlic

1 teaspoon salt

1/8 teaspoon ground black pepper

1 teaspoon Herbes de Provence

1/2 teaspoon red pepper flakes

2 tablespoons olive oil

1/2 cup water

2 tablespoons chopped parsley

Directions:

Take a saucepan, place it over medium-high heat, add oil and when hot, add onion, fennel, and garlic and cook for 20 minutes until softened.

Then add remaining ingredients except for olives and chickpeas, bring the mixture to boil, switch heat to medium-low level and simmer for 15 minutes.

Then add remaining ingredients, cook for 10 minutes until hot, garnish stew with parsley and serve.

Nutrition Value:

Calories: 395 Cal

Fat: 13 g

Carbs: 56 g

Protein: 16 g

Fiber: 13 g

Cabbage Stew

Preparation time: 10 minutes

Cooking time: 50 minutes

Servings: 6

Ingredients:

12 ounces cooked Cannellini beans

8 ounces smoked tofu, firm, sliced

1 medium cabbage, chopped

1 large white onion, peeled, julienned

2 ½ teaspoon minced garlic

1 tablespoon sweet paprika

5 tablespoons tomato paste

3 teaspoons smoked paprika

1/3 teaspoon ground black pepper

2 teaspoons dried thyme

2/3 teaspoon salt

½ tsp ground coriander

3 bay leaves

4 tablespoons olive oil

1 cup vegetable broth

Directions:

Take a large saucepan, place it over medium heat, add 3 tablespoons oil and when hot, add onion and garlic and cook for 3 minutes or until saute.

Add cabbage, pour in water, simmer for 10 minutes or until softened, then stir in all the spices and continue cooking for 30 minutes.

Add beans and tomato paste, pour in water, stir until mixed and cook for 15 minutes until thoroughly cooked.

Take a separate skillet pan, add 1 tablespoon oil and when hot, add tofu slices and cook for 5 minutes until golden brown on both sides.

Serve cooked cabbage stew with fried tofu.

Nutrition Value:

Calories: 182 Cal

Fat: 8.3 g

Carbs: 27 g

Protein: 5.5 g

Fiber: 9.4 g

Kimchi Stew

Preparation time: 10 minutes

Cooking time: 25 minutes

Servings: 4

Ingredients:

1 pound tofu, extra-firm, pressed, cut into 1-inch pieces

4 cups napa cabbage kimchi, vegan, chopped

1 small white onion, peeled, diced

2 cups sliced shiitake mushroom caps

1 ½ teaspoon minced garlic

2 tablespoons soy sauce

2 tablespoons olive oil, divided

4 cups vegetable broth

2 tablespoons chopped scallions

Directions:

Take a large pot, place it over medium heat, add 1 tablespoon oil and when hot, add tofu pieces in a single layer and cook for 10 minutes until browned on all sides.

When cooked, transfer tofu pieces to a plate, add remaining oil to the pot and when hot, add onion and cook for 5 minutes until soft.

Stir in garlic, cook for 1 minute until fragrant, stir in kimchi, continue cooking for 2 minutes, then add mushrooms and pour in broth.

Switch heat to medium-high level, bring the mixture to boil, then switch heat to medium-low level and simmer for 10 minutes until mushrooms are softened.

Stir in tofu, taste to adjust seasoning, and garnish with scallions.

Serve straight away.

Nutrition Value:

Calories: 153 Cal

Fat: 8.2 g

Carbs: 25 g

Protein: 8.4 g

Fiber: 2.6 g

African Peanut Lentil Soup

Preparation time: 10 minutes

Cooking time: 25 minutes

Servings: 3

Ingredients:

1/2 cup red lentils

1/2 medium white onion, sliced

2 medium tomatoes, chopped

1/2 cup baby spinach

1/2 cup sliced zucchini

1/2 cup sliced sweet potatoes

½ cup sliced potatoes

½ cup broccoli florets

2 teaspoons minced garlic

1 inch of ginger, grated

1 tablespoon tomato paste

1/4 teaspoon ground black pepper

1 teaspoon salt

1 ½ teaspoon ground cumin

2 teaspoons ground coriander

2 tablespoons peanuts

1 teaspoon Harissa Spice Blend

1 tablespoon sambal oelek

1/4 cup almond butter

1 teaspoon olive oil

1 teaspoon lemon juice

2 ½ cups vegetable stock

Directions:

Take a large saucepan, place it over medium heat, add oil and when hot, add onion and cook for 5 minutes until translucent.

Meanwhile, place tomatoes in a blender, add garlic, ginger and sambal oelek along with all the spices and pulse until pureed.

Pour this mixture into the onions, cook for 5 minutes, then add remaining ingredients except for spinach, peanuts and lemon juice and simmer for 15 minutes.

Taste to adjust the seasoning, stir in spinach, and cook for 5 minutes until cooked.

Ladle soup into bowls, garnish with lime juice and peanuts and serve.

Nutrition Value:

Calories: 411 Cal

Fat: 17 g

Carbs: 50 g

Protein: 20 g

Fiber: 18 g

Spicy Bean Stew

Preparation time: 5 minutes

Cooking time: 50 minutes

Servings: 4

Ingredients:

7 ounces cooked black eye beans

14 ounces chopped tomatoes

2 medium carrots, peeled, diced

7 ounces cooked kidney beans

1 leek, diced

½ a chili, chopped

1 teaspoon minced garlic

1/3 teaspoon ground black pepper

2/3 teaspoon salt

1 teaspoon red chili powder

1 lemon, juiced

3 tablespoons white wine

1 tablespoon olive oil

1 2/3 cups vegetable stock

Directions:

Take a large saucepan, place it over medium-high heat, add oil and when hot, add leeks and cook for 8 minutes or until softened.

Then add carrots, continue cooking for 4 minutes, stir in chili and garlic, pour in the wine, and continue cooking for 2 minutes.

Add tomatoes, stir in lemon juice, pour in the stock and bring the mixture to boil.

Switch heat to medium level, simmer for 35 minutes until stew has thickened, then add both beans along with remaining ingredients and cook for 5 minutes until hot.

Serve straight away.

Nutrition Value:

Calories: 114 Cal

Fat: 1.6 g

Carbs: 19 g

Protein: 6 g

Fiber: 8.4 g

Eggplant, Onion and Tomato Stew

Preparation time: 5 minutes

Cooking time: 5 minutes

Servings: 4

Ingredients:

3 1/2 cups cubed eggplant

1 cup diced white onion

2 cups diced tomatoes

1 teaspoon ground cumin

1/8 teaspoon ground cayenne pepper

1 teaspoon salt

1 cup tomato sauce

1/2 cup water

Directions:

Switch on the instant pot, place all the ingredients in it, stir until mixed, and seal the pot.

Press the 'manual' button and cook for 5 minutes at high-pressure setting until cooked.

When done, do quick pressure release, open the instant pot, and stir the stew.

Serve straight away.

Nutrition Value:

Calories: 88 Cal

Fat: 1 g

Carbs: 21 g

Protein: 3 g

Fiber: 6 g

White Bean Stew

Preparation time: 5 minutes

Cooking time: 10 hours and 10 minutes

Servings: 10

Ingredients:

2 cups chopped spinach

28 ounces diced tomatoes

2 pounds white beans, dried

2 cups chopped chard

2 large carrots, peeled, diced

2 cups chopped kale

3 large celery stalks, diced

1 medium white onion, peeled, diced

1 ½ teaspoon minced garlic

2 tablespoons salt

1 teaspoon dried rosemary

½ teaspoon Ground black pepper, to taste

1 teaspoon dried thyme

1 teaspoon dried oregano

1 bay leaf

10 cups water

Directions:

Switch on the slow cooker, add all the ingredients in it, except for kale, chard, and spinach and stir until combined.

Shut the cooker with lid and cook for 10 hours at a low heat setting until thoroughly cooked.

When done, stir in kale, chard, and spinach, and cook for 10 minutes until leaves wilt.

Serve straight away.

Nutrition Value:

Calories: 109 Cal

Fat: 2.4 g

Carbs: 17.8 g

Protein: 5.3 g

Fiber: 6 g

Brussel Sprouts Stew

Preparation time: 10 minutes

Cooking time: 55 minutes

Servings: 4

Ingredients:

35 ounces Brussels sprouts

5 medium potato, peeled, chopped

1 medium onion, peeled, chopped

2 carrot, peeled, cubed

2 teaspoon smoked paprika

1/8 teaspoon ground black pepper

1/8 teaspoon salt

3 tablespoons caraway seeds

1/2 teaspoon red chili powder

1 tablespoon nutmeg

1 tablespoon olive oil

4 ½ cups hot vegetable stock

Directions:

Take a large pot, place it over medium-high heat, add oil and when hot, add onion and cook for 1 minute.

Then add carrot and potato, cook for 2 minutes, then add Brussel sprouts and cook for 5 minutes.

Stir in all the spices, pour in vegetable stock, bring the mixture to boil, switch heat to medium-low and simmer for 45 minutes until cooked and stew reach to desired thickness.

Serve straight away.

Nutrition Value:

Calories: 156 Cal

Fat: 3 g

Carbs: 22 g

Protein: 12 g

Fiber: 5.1100 g

Vegetarian Gumbo

Preparation time: 10 minutes

Cooking time: 45 minutes

Servings: 4

Ingredients:

1 1/2 cups diced zucchini

16-ounces cooked red beans

4 cups sliced okra

1 1/2 cups diced green pepper

1 1/2 cups chopped white onion

1 1/2 cups diced red bell pepper

8 cremini mushrooms, quartered

1 cup sliced celery

3 teaspoons minced garlic

1 medium tomato, chopped

1 teaspoon red pepper flakes

1 teaspoon dried thyme

3 tablespoons all-purpose flour

1 tablespoon smoked paprika

1 teaspoon dried oregano

1/4 teaspoon nutmeg

1 teaspoon soy sauce

1 1/2 teaspoons liquid smoke

2 tablespoons mustard

1 tablespoon apple cider vinegar

1 tablespoon Worcestershire sauce, vegetarian

1/2 teaspoon hot sauce

3 tablespoons olive oil

4 cups vegetable stock

1/2 cups sliced green onion

4 cups cooked jasmine rice

Directions:

Take a Dutch oven, place it over medium heat, add oil and flour and cook for 5 minutes until fragrant.

Switch heat to the medium low level, and continue cooking for 20 minutes until roux becomes dark brown, whisking constantly.

Meanwhile, place the tomato in a food processor, add garlic and onion along with remaining ingredients, except for stock, zucchini, celery, mushroom, green and red bell pepper, and pulse for 2 minutes until smooth.

Pour the mixture into the pan, return pan over medium-high heat, stir until mixed, and cook for 5 minutes until all the liquid has evaporated.

Stir in stock, bring it to simmer, then add remaining vegetables and simmer for 20 minutes until tender.

Garnish gumbo with green onions and serve with rice.

Nutrition Value:

Calories: 160 Cal

Fat: 7.3 g

Carbs: 20 g

Protein: 7 g

Fiber: 5.7 g

Black Bean and Quinoa Stew

Preparation time: 10 minutes

Cooking time: 6 hours

Servings: 6

Ingredients:

1 pound black beans, dried, soaked overnight

3/4 cup quinoa, uncooked

1 medium red bell pepper, cored, chopped

1 medium red onion, peeled, diced

1 medium green bell pepper, cored, chopped

28-ounce diced tomatoes

2 dried chipotle peppers

1 ½ teaspoon minced garlic

2/3 teaspoon sea salt

2 teaspoons red chili powder

1/3 teaspoon ground black pepper

1 teaspoon coriander powder

1 dried cinnamon stick

1/4 cup cilantro

7 cups of water

Directions:

Switch on the slow cooker, add all the ingredients in it, except for salt, and stir until mixed.

Shut the cooker with lid and cook for 6 hours at a high heat setting until cooked.

When done, stir salt into the stew until mixed, remove cinnamon sticks and serve.

Nutrition Value:

Calories: 308 Cal

Fat: 2 g

Carbs: 70 g

Protein: 23 g

Fiber: 32 g

Root Vegetable Stew

Preparation time: 10 minutes

Cooking time: 8 hours and 10 minutes

Servings: 6

Ingredients:

2 cups chopped kale

1 large white onion, peeled, chopped

1 pound parsnips, peeled, chopped

1 pound potatoes, peeled, chopped

2 celery ribs, chopped

1 pound butternut squash, peeled, deseeded, chopped

1 pound carrots, peeled, chopped

3 teaspoons minced garlic

1 pound sweet potatoes, peeled, chopped

1 bay leaf

1 teaspoon ground black pepper

1/2 teaspoon sea salt

1 tablespoon chopped sage

3 cups vegetable broth

Directions:

Switch on the slow cooker, add all the ingredients in it, except for the kale, and stir until mixed.

Shut the cooker with lid and cook for 8 hours at a low heat setting until cooked.

When done, add kale into the stew, stir until mixed, and cook for 10 minutes until leaves have wilted.

Serve straight away.

Nutrition Value:

Calories: 120 Cal

Fat: 1 g

Carbs: 28 g

Protein: 4 g

Fiber: 6 g

Portobello Mushroom Stew

Preparation time: 10 minutes

Cooking time: 8 hours

Servings: 4

Ingredients:

8 cups vegetable broth

1 cup dried wild mushrooms

1 cup dried chickpeas

3 cups chopped potato

2 cups chopped carrots

1 cup corn kernels

2 cups diced white onions

1 tablespoon minced parsley

3 cups chopped zucchini

1 tablespoon minced rosemary

1 1/2 teaspoon ground black pepper

1 teaspoon dried sage

2/3 teaspoon salt

1 teaspoon dried oregano

3 tablespoons soy sauce

1 1/2 teaspoons liquid smoke

8 ounces tomato paste

Directions:

Switch on the slow cooker, add all the ingredients in it, and stir until mixed.

Shut the cooker with lid and cook for 10 hours at a high heat setting until cooked.

Serve straight away.

Nutrition Value:

Calories: 447 Cal

Fat: 36 g

Carbs: 24 g

Protein: 11 g

Fiber: 2 g

Chapter 4. Beans and Grains

Garlic and White Bean Soup

Cooking time: 10 minutes

Servings: 4

Ingredients:

45 ounces cooked cannellini beans

1/4 teaspoon dried thyme

2 teaspoons minced garlic

1/8 teaspoon crushed red pepper

1/2 teaspoon dried rosemary

1/8 teaspoon ground black pepper

2 tablespoons olive oil

4 cups vegetable broth

Directions:

Place one-third of white beans in a food processor, then pour in 2 cups broth and pulse for 2 minutes until smooth.

Place a pot over medium heat, add oil and when hot, add garlic and cook for 1 minute until fragrant.

Add pureed beans into the pan along with remaining beans, sprinkle with spices and herbs, pour in the broth, stir until combined, and bring the mixture to boil over medium-high heat.

Switch heat to medium-low level, simmer the beans for 15 minutes, and then mash them with a fork.

Taste the soup to adjust seasoning and then serve.

Nutrition:

Calories: 222 Cal

Fat: 7 g

Carbs: 13 g

Protein: 11.2 g

Fiber: 9.1 g

Coconut Curry Lentils

Preparation time: 10 minutes

Cooking time: 40 minutes

Servings: 4

Ingredients:

1 cup brown lentils

1 small white onion, peeled, chopped

1 teaspoon minced garlic

1 teaspoon grated ginger

3 cups baby spinach

1 tablespoon curry powder

2 tablespoons olive oil

13 ounces coconut milk, unsweetened

2 cups vegetable broth

For Serving:

4 cups cooked rice

1/4 cup chopped cilantro

Directions:

Place a large pot over medium heat, add oil and when hot, add ginger and garlic and cook for 1 minute until fragrant.

Add onion, cook for 5 minutes, stir in curry powder, cook for 1 minute until toasted, add lentils and pour in broth.

Switch heat to medium-high level, bring the mixture to a boil, then switch heat to the low level and simmer for 20 minutes until tender and all the liquid is absorbed.

Pour in milk, stir until combined, turn heat to medium level, and simmer for 10 minutes until thickened.

Then remove the pot from heat, stir in spinach, let it stand for 5 minutes until its leaves wilts and then top with cilantro.

Serve lentils with rice.

Nutrition:

Calories: 184 Cal

Fat: 3.7 g

Carbs: 30 g

Protein: 11.3 g

Fiber: 10.7 g

Tomato, Kale, and White Bean Skillet

Preparation time: 10 minutes

Cooking time: 10 minutes

Servings: 4

Ingredients:

30 ounces cooked cannellini beans

3.5 ounces sun-dried tomatoes, packed in oil, chopped

6 ounces kale, chopped

1 teaspoon minced garlic

1/4 teaspoon ground black pepper

1/4 teaspoon salt

1/2 tablespoon dried basil

1/8 teaspoon red pepper flakes

1 tablespoon apple cider vinegar

1 tablespoon olive oil

2 tablespoons oil from sun-dried tomatoes

Directions:

Prepare the dressing and for this, place basil, black pepper, salt, vinegar, and red pepper flakes in a small bowl, add oil from sun-dried tomatoes and whisk until combined.

Take a skillet pan, place it over medium heat, add olive oil and when hot, add garlic and cook for 1 minute until fragrant.

Add kale, splash with some water and cook for 3 minutes until kale leaves have wilted.

Add tomatoes and beans, stir well and cook for 3 minutes until heated.

Remove pan from heat, drizzle with the prepared dressing, toss until mixed and serve.

Nutrition:

Calories: 264 Cal

Fat: 12 g

Carbs: 38 g

Protein: 9 g

Fiber: 13 g

Chard Wraps With Millet

Preparation time: 25 minutes

Cooking time: 0 minute

Servings: 4

Ingredients:

1 carrot, cut into ribbons

1/2 cup millet, cooked

1/2 of a large cucumber, cut into ribbons

1/2 cup chickpeas, cooked

1 cup sliced cabbage

1/3 cup hummus

Mint leaves as needed for topping

Hemp seeds as needed for topping

1 bunch of Swiss rainbow chard

Directions:

Spread hummus on one side of chard, place some of millet, vegetables, and chickpeas on it, sprinkle with some mint leaves and hemp seeds and wrap it like a burrito.

Serve straight away.

Nutrition:

Calories: 152 Cal

Fat: 4.5 g

Carbs: 25 g

Protein: 3.5 g

Fiber: 2.4 g

Quinoa Meatballs

Preparation time: 10 minutes

Cooking time: 35 minutes

Servings: 4

Ingredients:

1 cup quinoa, cooked

1 tablespoon flax meal

1 cup diced white onion

1 ½ teaspoon minced garlic

1/2 teaspoon salt

1 teaspoon dried oregano

1 teaspoon lemon zest

1 teaspoon paprika

1 teaspoon dried basil

3 tablespoons water

2 tablespoons olive oil

1 cup grated vegan mozzarella cheese

Marinara sauce as needed for serving

Directions:

Place flax meal in a bowl, stir in water and set aside until required.

Take a large skillet pan, place it over medium heat, add 1 tablespoon oil and when hot, add onion and cook for 2 minutes.

Stir in all the spices and herbs, then stir in quinoa until combined and cook for 2 minutes.

Transfer quinoa mixture in a bowl, add flax meal mixture, lemon zest, and cheese, stir until well mixed and then shape the mixture into twelve 1 ½ inch balls.

Arrange balls on a baking sheet lined with parchment paper, refrigerate the balls for 30 minutes and then bake for 20 minutes at 400 degrees F.

Serve balls with marinara sauce.

Nutrition:

Calories: 100 Cal

Fat: 100 g

Carbs: 100 g

Protein: 100 g

Fiber: 100 g

Rice Stuffed Jalapeños

Preparation time: 5 minutes

Cooking time: 15 minutes

Servings: 6

Ingredients:

3 medium-sized potatoes, peeled, cubed, boiled

2 large carrots, peeled, chopped, boiled

3 tablespoons water

1/4 teaspoon onion powder

1 teaspoons salt

1/2 cup nutritional yeast

1/4 teaspoon garlic powder

1 lime, juiced

3 tablespoons water

Cooked rice as needed

3 jalapeños pepper, halved

1 red bell pepper, sliced, for garnish

½ cup vegetable broth

Directions:

Place boiled vegetables in a food processor, pour in broth and pulse until smooth.

Add garlic powder, onion powder, salt, water, and lime juice, pulse until combined, then add yeast and blend until smooth.

Tip the mixture in a bowl, add rice, and stir until incorporated.

Cut each jalapeno into half lengthwise, brush them with oil, season them with some salt, stuff them with rice mixture and bake them for 20 minutes at 400 degrees F until done.

Serve straight away.

Nutrition:

Calories: 148 Cal

Fat: 3.7 g

Carbs: 12.2 g

Protein: 2 g

Fiber: 2 g

Pineapple Fried Rice

Preparation time: 5 minutes

Cooking time: 12 minutes

Servings: 2

Ingredients:

2 cups brown rice, cooked

1/2 cup sunflower seeds, toasted

2/3 cup green peas

1 teaspoon minced garlic

1 large red bell pepper, cored, diced

1 tablespoon grated ginger

2/3 cup pineapple chunks with juice

2 tablespoons coconut oil

1 bunch of green onions, sliced

For the Sauce:

4 tablespoons soy sauce

1/2 cup pineapple juice

1/2 teaspoon sesame oil

1/2 a lime, juiced

Directions:

Take a skillet pan, place it over medium-high heat, add oil and when hot, add red bell pepper, pineapple pieces, and two-third of onion, cook for 5 minutes, then stir in ginger and garlic and cook for 1 minute.

Switch heat to the high level, add rice to the pan, stir until combined and cook for 5 minutes.

When done, fold in sunflower seeds and peas and set aside until required.

Prepare the sauce and for this, place sesame oil in a small bowl, add soy sauce and pineapple juice and whisk until combined.

Drizzle sauce over rice, drizzle with lime juice, and serve straight away.

Nutrition:

Calories: 179 Cal

Fat: 5.5 g

Carbs: 30 g

Protein: 3.3 g

Fiber: 2 g

Lentil and Wild Rice Soup

Preparation time: 10 minutes

Cooking time: 40 minutes

Servings: 4

Ingredients:

1/2 cup cooked mixed beans

12 ounces cooked lentils

2 stalks of celery, sliced

1 1/2 cup mixed wild rice, cooked

1 large sweet potato, peeled, chopped

1/2 medium butternut, peeled, chopped

4 medium carrots, peeled, sliced

1 medium onion, peeled, diced

10 cherry tomatoes

1/2 red chili, deseeded, diced

1 ½ teaspoon minced garlic

1/2 teaspoon salt

2 teaspoons mixed dried herbs

1 teaspoon coconut oil

2 cups vegetable broth

Directions:

Take a large pot, place it over medium-high heat, add oil and when it melts, add onion and cook for 5 minutes.

Stir in garlic and chili, cook for 3 minutes, then add remaining vegetables, pour in the broth, stir and bring the mixture to a boil.

Switch heat to medium-low heat, cook the soup for 20 minutes, then stir in remaining ingredients and continue cooking for 10 minutes until soup has reached to desired thickness.

Serve straight away.

Nutrition:

Calories: 331 Cal

Fat: 2 g

Carbs: 54 g

Protein: 13 g

Fiber: 12 g

Black Bean Meatball Salad

Preparation time: 10 minutes

Cooking time: 25 minutes

Servings: 4

Ingredients:

For the Meatballs:

1/2 cup quinoa, cooked

1 cup cooked black beans

3 cloves of garlic, peeled

1 small red onion, peeled

1 teaspoon ground dried coriander

1 teaspoon ground dried cumin

1 teaspoon smoked paprika

For the Salad:

1 large sweet potato, peeled, diced

1 lemon, juiced

1 teaspoon minced garlic

1 cup coriander leaves

1/3 cup almonds

1/3 teaspoon ground black pepper

½ teaspoon salt

1 1/2 tablespoons olive oil

Directions:

Prepare the meatballs and for this, place beans and puree in a blender, pulse until pureed, and this place this mixture in a medium bowl.

Add onion and garlic, process until chopped, add to the bean mixture, add all the spices, stir until combined, and shape the mixture into uniform balls.

Bake the balls on a greased baking sheet for 25 minutes at 350 degrees F until browned.

Meanwhile, spread sweet potatoes on a baking sheet lined with baking paper, drizzle with ½ tablespoon oil, toss until coated and bake for 20 minutes with the meatballs.

Prepare the dressing, and for this, place remaining ingredients for the salad in a food processor and pulse until smooth.

Place roasted sweet potatoes in a bowl, drizzle with the dressing, toss until coated, and then top with meatballs.

Serve straight away.

Nutrition:

Calories: 140 Cal

Fat: 8 g

Carbs: 8 g

Protein: 10 g

Fiber: 4 g

Black Beans and Cauliflower Rice

Preparation time: 10 minutes

Cooking time: 20 minutes

Servings: 4

Ingredients:

3 cups cauliflower rice

15.5 ounces cooked black beans

1/2 cup diced red bell pepper

1/2 cup chopped onion

3 tablespoons chopped pickled jalapeno

1 ½ teaspoon minced garlic

¼ teaspoon ground black pepper

1/3 teaspoon sea salt

1/4 teaspoon ground cayenne pepper

2 tablespoons olive oil

1/2 cup diced parsley

Directions:

Take a large skillet pan, place it over medium heat, add oil and garlic and cook for 2 minutes.

Then add onion and bell pepper, season with black pepper, salt, and cayenne pepper, cook for 5 minutes, then stir in jalapeno pepper and top with cauliflower rice.

Season with salt and black pepper, cook for 7 minutes, turning halfway, then add beans and cook for 2 minutes until hot.

Garnish with parsley and serve.

Nutrition:

Calories: 270.3 Cal

Fat: 1.6 g

Carbs: 52.7 g

Protein: 13.5 g

Fiber: 13.1 g

Black Bean Stuffed Sweet Potatoes

Preparation time: 15 minutes

Cooking time: 65 minutes

Servings: 4

Ingredients:

4 large sweet potatoes

15 ounces cooked black beans

1/2 teaspoon ground black pepper

1/2 of a medium red onion, peeled, diced

1/2 teaspoon sea salt

1/4 teaspoon onion powder

1/4 teaspoon garlic powder

1/4 teaspoon red chili powder

1/4 teaspoon cumin

1 teaspoon lime juice

1 1/2 tablespoons olive oil

1/2 cup cashew cream sauce

Directions:

Spread sweet potatoes on a baking tray greased with oil and bake for 65 minutes at 350 degrees F until tender.

Meanwhile, prepare the sauce, and for this, whisk together the cream sauce, black pepper and lime juice until combined, set aside until required.

When 10 minutes of the baking time of potatoes are left, heat a skillet pan with oil, then add onion and cook for 5 minutes until golden.

Then stir in spice, cook for another 3 minutes, stir in bean until combined and cook for 5 minutes until hot.

Let roasted sweet potatoes cool for 10 minutes, then cut them open, mash the flesh and top with bean mixture, cilantro and avocado, and then drizzle with cream sauce.

Serve straight away.

Nutrition:

Calories: 387 Cal

Fat: 16.1 g

Carbs: 53 g

Protein: 10.4 g

Fiber: 17.6 g

Black Bean and Quinoa Salad

Preparation time: 10 minutes

Cooking time: 0 minute

Servings: 10

Ingredients:

15 ounces cooked black beans

1 medium red bell pepper, cored, chopped

1 cup quinoa, cooked

1 medium green bell pepper, cored, chopped

1/2 cup vegan feta cheese, crumbled

Directions:

Place all the ingredients in a large bowl, except for cheese, and stir until incorporated.

Top the salad with cheese and serve straight away.

Nutrition:

Calories: 64 Cal

Fat: 1 g

Carbs: 8 g

Protein: 3 g

Fiber: 3 g

Chickpea Fajitas

Preparation time: 10 minutes

Cooking time: 30 minutes

Servings: 4

Ingredients:

For the Chickpea Fajitas:

1 1/2 cups cooked chickpeas

1 medium white onion, peeled, sliced

2 medium green bell peppers, cored, sliced

1 tablespoon fajita seasoning

2 tablespoons olive oil

For the Cream:

1/2 cup cashews, soaked

1 clove of garlic, peeled

½ teaspoon salt

1/2 teaspoon ground cumin

1/4 cup lime juice

1/4 cup water

1 tablespoon olive oil

To serve:

Sliced avocado for topping

Chopped lettuce for topping

4 flour tortillas

Chopped tomatoes for topping

Salsa for topping

Chopped cilantro for topping

Directions:

Prepare chickpeas and for this, whisk together seasoning and oil until combined, add onion, pepper, and chickpeas, toss until well coated, then spread them in a baking sheet and roast for 30 minutes at 400 degrees F until crispy and browned, stirring halfway.

Meanwhile, prepare the cream and for this, place all of its ingredients in a food processor and pulse until smooth, set aside until required.

When chickpeas and vegetables have roasted, top them evenly on tortillas, then top them evenly with avocado, lettuce, tomatoes, salsa, and cilantro and serve.

Nutrition:

Calories: 391 Cal

Fat: 16 g

Carbs: 43 g

Protein: 8 g

Fiber: 9 g

Coconut Chickpea Curry

Preparation time: 10 minutes

Cooking time: 30 minutes

Servings: 4

Ingredients:

2 teaspoons coconut flour

16 ounces cooked chickpeas

14 ounces tomatoes, diced

1 large red onion, sliced

1 ½ teaspoon minced garlic

½ teaspoon of sea salt

1 teaspoon curry powder

1/3 teaspoon ground black pepper

1 ½ tablespoons garam masala

1/4 teaspoon cumin

1 small lime, juiced

13.5 ounces coconut milk, unsweetened

2 tablespoons coconut oil

Directions:

Take a large pot, place it over medium-high heat, add oil and when it melts, add onions and tomatoes, season with salt and black pepper and cook for 5 minutes.

Switch heat to medium-low level, cook for 10 minutes until tomatoes have released their liquid, then add chickpeas and stir in garlic, curry powder, garam masala, and cumin until combined.

Stir in milk and flour, bring the mixture to boil, then switch heat to medium heat and simmer the curry for 12 minutes until cooked.

Taste to adjust seasoning, drizzle with lime juice, and serve.

Nutrition:

Calories: 225 Cal

Fat: 9.4 g

Carbs: 28.5 g

Protein: 7.3 g

Fiber: 9 g

Mediterranean Chickpea Casserole

Preparation time: 10 minutes

Cooking time: 60 minutes

Servings: 4

Ingredients:

3 cups baby spinach

2 medium red onions, peeled, diced

2 1/2 cups tomatoes

3 cups cooked chickpeas

1 ½ teaspoon minced garlic

1/3 teaspoon ground black pepper

1 ¼ teaspoon salt

1/4 teaspoon allspice

1 tablespoon coconut sugar

1 teaspoon dried oregano

1/4 teaspoon cayenne

1/4 teaspoon cloves

2 bay leaves

1 tablespoon coconut oil

2 tablespoons olive oil

1 cup vegetable stock

1 lemon, juiced

2 ounces vegan feta cheese

Directions:

Take a large skillet pan, place it over medium-high heat, add coconut oil and when it melts, add onion and cook for 5 minutes until softened.

Switch heat to medium-low level, stir in garlic, cook for 2 minutes, then stir in tomatoes, add all the spices and bay leaves, pour in the stock, stir until mixed and cook for 20 minutes.

Then stir in chickpeas, simmer cooking for 15 minutes until the cooking liquid has reduced by one-third, stir in spinach and cook for 3 minutes until it begins to wilt.

Then stir in olive oil, sugar and lemon juice, taste to adjust seasoning, and remove and discard bay leaves.

When done, top chickpeas with cheese, broil for 5 minutes until cheese has melted and golden brown, then garnish with parsley and serve.

Nutrition:

Calories: 257.8 Cal

Fat: 3.8 g

Carbs: 47.1 g

Protein: 10.3 g

Fiber: 9.4 g

Zoodles with White Beans

Preparation time: 10 minutes

Cooking time: 20 minutes

Servings: 4

Ingredients:

15 ounces cooked cannellini beans

2 medium zucchini, spiralized into noodles

3 teaspoons minced garlic

1 cup chopped Roma tomatoes

2/3 teaspoon salt

1/8 teaspoon red pepper flakes

1/4 cup olive oil

1/4 cup chopped parsley

4 ounces whole-grain spaghetti, cooked

Directions:

Cook the pasta, drain it, transfer it into a bowl, add zucchini noodles and toss until mixed.

Take a pot, place it over low heat, add oil, garlic, and red pepper flakes, stir until cook for 5 minutes until garlic is golden brown.

Then add all the ingredients, except for parsley and salt, toss until mixed and cook for 5 minutes until thoroughly heated.

When done, season with salt, top with parsley and serve.

Nutrition:

Calories: 301 Cal

Fat: 15 g

Carbs: 34 g

Protein: 11 g

Fiber: 7 g

Sweet Potato and White Bean Skillet

Preparation time: 10 minutes

Cooking time: 45 minutes

Servings: 4

Ingredients:

1 large bunch of kale, chopped

2 large sweet potatoes, peeled, ¼-inch cubes

12 ounces cannellini beans

1 small onion, peeled, diced

1/8 teaspoon red pepper flakes

1 teaspoon salt

1 teaspoon cumin

½ teaspoon ground black pepper

1 teaspoon curry powder

1 1/2 tablespoons coconut oil

6 ounces coconut milk, unsweetened

Directions:

Take a large skillet pan, place it over medium heat, add ½ tablespoon oil and when it melts, add onion and cook for 5 minutes.

Then stir in sweet potatoes, stir well, cook for 5 minutes, then season with all the spices, cook for 1 minute and remove the pan from heat.

Take another pan, add remaining oil in it, place it over medium heat and when oil melts, add kale, season with some salt and black pepper, stir well, pour in the milk and cook for 15 minutes until tender.

Then add beans, beans, and red pepper, stir until mixed and cook for 5 minutes until hot.

Serve straight away.

Nutrition:

Calories: 263 Cal

Fat: 4 g

Carbs: 44 g

Protein: 13 g

Fiber: 12 g

Cauliflower & Apple Salad

Servings: 4

Preparation Time: 25 Minutes

Calories: 198

Protein: 7 Grams

Fat: 8 Grams

Carbs: 32 Grams

Ingredients:

3 Cups Cauliflower, Chopped into Florets

2 Cups Baby Kale

1 Sweet Apple, Cored & Chopped

¼ Cup Basil, Fresh & Chopped

¼ Cup Mint, Fresh & Chopped

¼ Cup Parsley, Fresh & Chopped

1/3 Cup Scallions, Sliced Thin

2 Tablespoons Yellow Raisins

1 Tablespoon Sun Dried Tomatoes, Chopped

½ Cup Miso Dressing, Optional

¼ Cup Roasted Pumpkin Seeds, Optional

Directions:

Combine everything together, tossing before serving.

Corn & Black Bean Salad

Salad: 6

Preparation Time: 10 Minutes

Calories: 159

Protein: 6.4 Grams

Fat: 5.6 Grams

Carbs: 23.7 Grams

Ingredients:

¼ Cup Cilantro, Fresh & Chopped

1 Can Corn, Drained (10 Ounces)

1/8 Cup Red Onion, Chopped

1 Can Black Beans, Drained (15 Ounces)

1 Tomato, Chopped

3 Tablespoons Lemon Juice, Fresh

2 Tablespoons Olive Oil

Sea Salt & Black Pepper to Taste

Directions:

Mix everything together, and then refrigerate until cool. Serve cold.

Spinach & Orange Salad

Servings: 6

Preparation Time: 15 Minutes

Calories: 99

Protein: 2.5 Grams

Fat: 5 Grams

Carbs: 13.1 Grams

Ingredients:

¼ -1/3 Cup Vegan Dressing

3 Oranges, Medium, Peeled, Seeded & Sectioned

¾ lb. Spinach, Fresh & Torn

1 Red Onion, Medium, Sliced & Separated into Rings

Directions:

Toss everything together, and serve with dressing.

Red Pepper & Broccoli Salad

Servings: 2

Preparation Time: 15 Minutes

Calories: 185

Protein: 4 Grams

Fat: 14 Grams

Carbs: 8 Grams

Ingredients:

Ounces Lettuce Salad Mix

1 Head Broccoli, Chopped into Florets

1 Red Pepper, Seeded & Chopped

Dressing:

3 Tablespoons White Wine Vinegar

1 Teaspoon Dijon Mustard

1 Clove Garlic, Peeled & Chopped Fine

½ Teaspoon Black Pepper

½ Teaspoon Sea Salt, Fine

2 Tablespoons Olive Oil

1 Tablespoon Parsley, Chopped

Directions:

In boiling water, drain the broccoli it on a paper towel.

Whisk together all dressing ingredients.

Toss ingredients together before serving.

Lentil Potato Salad

Servings: 2

Preparation Time: 35 Minutes

Calories: 400

Protein: 7 Grams

Fat: 26 Grams

Carbs: 39 Grams

Ingredients:

½ Cup Beluga Lentils

8 Fingerling Potatoes

1 Cup Scallions, Sliced Thin

¼ Cup Cherry Tomatoes, Halved

¼ Cup Lemon Vinaigrette

Sea Salt & Black Pepper to Taste

Directions:

Bring two cups of water to simmer in a pot, adding your lentils. Cook for twenty to twenty-five minutes, and then drain. Your lentils should be tender.

Reduce to a simmer, cooking for fifteen minutes, and then drain. Halve your potatoes once they're cool enough to touch.

Put your lentils on a serving plate, and then top with scallions, potatoes and tomatoes. Drizzle with your vinaigrette, and season with salt and pepper.

Black Bean & Corn Salad with Avocado

Preparation Time: 20 minutes

Servings: 6

Ingredients:

1 and ½ cups corn kernels, cooked & frozen or canned

½ cup olive oil

1 minced clove garlic

⅓ cup lime juice, fresh

1 avocado (peeled, pitted & diced)

⅛ tsp. cayenne pepper

2 cans black beans, (approximately 15 oz.)

6 thinly sliced green onions

½ cup chopped cilantro, fresh

2 chopped tomatoes

1 chopped red bell pepper

Chili powder

½ tsp. salt

Directions:

In a small jar, place the olive oil, lime juice, garlic, cayenne, and salt.

Cover with lid; shake until all the ingredients under the jar are mixed well.

Toss the green onions, corn, beans, bell pepper, avocado, tomatoes, and cilantro together in a large bowl or plastic container with a cover.

Shake the lime dressing for a second time and transfer it over the salad ingredients.

Stir salad to coat the beans and vegetables with the dressing; cover & refrigerate.

To blend the flavors completely, let this sit a moment or two.

Remove the container from the refrigerator from time to time; turn upside down & back gently a couple of times to reorganize the dressing.

Nutrition: 448 Calories, 24.3 g Total Fat, 0 mg Cholesterol, 50.8 g Total Carbohydrate, 14.3 g Dietary Fiber, 13.2 g Protein

Summer Chickpea Salad

Servings: 4

Preparation Time: 15 Minutes

Calories: 145

Protein: 4 Grams

Fat: 7.5 Grams

Carbs: 16 Grams

Ingredients:

1 ½ Cups Cherry Tomatoes, Halved

1 Cup English Cucumber, Slices

1 Cup Chickpeas, Canned, Unsalted, Drained & Rinsed

¼ Cup Red Onion, Slivered

2 Tablespoon Olive Oil

1 ½ Tablespoons Lemon Juice, Fresh

1 ½ Tablespoons Lemon Juice, Fresh

Sea Salt & Black Pepper to Taste

Directions:

Mix everything together, and toss to combine before serving.

Edamame Salad

Servings: 1

Preparation Time: 15 Minutes

Calories: 299

Protein: 20 Grams

Fat: 9 Grams

Carbs: 38 Grams

Ingredients:

¼ Cup Red Onion, Chopped

1 Cup Corn Kernels, Fresh

1 Cup Edamame Beans, Shelled & Thawed

1 Red Bell Pepper, Chopped

2-3 Tablespoons Lime Juice, Fresh

5-6 Basil Leaves, Fresh & Sliced

5-6 Mint Leaves, Fresh & Sliced

Sea Salt & Black Pepper to Taste

Directions:

Place everything into a Mason jar, and then seal the jar tightly. Shake well before serving.

Fruity Kale Salad

Servings: 4

Preparation Time: 30 Minutes

Calories: 220

Protein: 4 Grams

Fat: 17 Grams

Carbs: 16 Grams

Ingredients:

Salad:

10 Ounces Baby Kale

½ Cup Pomegranate Arils

1 Tablespoon Olive Oil

1 Apple, Sliced

Dressing:

3 Tablespoons Apple Cider Vinegar

3 Tablespoons Olive Oil

1 Tablespoon Tahini Sauce (Optional)

Sea Salt & Black Pepper to Taste

Directions:

Wash and dry the kale. If kale is too expensive, you can also use lettuce, arugula or spinach. Take the stems out, and chop it.

Combine all of your salad ingredients together.

Combine all of your dressing ingredients together before drizzling it over the salad to serve.

Olive & Fennel Salad

Servings: 3

Preparation Time: 5 Minutes

Calories: 331

Protein: 3 Grams

Fat: 29 Grams

Carbs: 15 Grams

Ingredients:

6 Tablespoons Olive Oil

3 Fennel Bulbs, Trimmed, Cored & Quartered

2 Tablespoons Parsley, Fresh & Chopped

1 Lemon, Juiced & Zested

12 Black Olives

Sea Salt & Black Pepper to Taste

Directions:

Grease your baking dish, and then place your fennel in it. Make sure the cut side is up.

Mix your lemon zest, lemon juice, salt, pepper and oil, pouring it over your fennel.

Sprinkle your olives over it, and bake at 400.

Serve with parsley.

Avocado & Radish Salad

Servings: 2

Preparation Time: 10 Minutes

Calories: 223

Protein: 3 Grams

Fat: 19 Grams

Carbs: 10 Grams

Ingredients:

1 Avocado, Sliced

6 Radishes, Sliced

2 Tomatoes, Sliced

1 Lettuce Head, Leaves Separated

½ Red Onion, Peeled & Sliced

Dressing:

½ Cup Olive Oil

¼ Cup Lime Juice, Fresh

¼ Cup Apple Cider Vinegar

3 Cloves Garlic, Chopped Fine

Sea Salt & Black Pepper to Taste

Directions:

Spread your lettuce leaves on a platter, and then layer with your onion, tomatoes, avocado and radishes.

Whisk your dressing ingredients together before drizzling it over your salad.

Zucchini & Lemon Salad

Servings: 2

Preparation Time: 3 Hours 10 Minutes

Calories: 159

Protein: 3 Grams

Fat: 14 Grams

Net Carbs: 7 Grams

Ingredients:

1 Green Zucchini, Sliced into Rounds

1 Yellow Squash, Zucchini, Sliced into Rounds

1 Clove Garlic, Peeled & Chopped

2 Tablespoons Olive Oil

2 Tablespoons Basil, Fresh

1 Lemon, Juiced & Zested

¼ Cup Coconut Milk

Sea Salt & Black Pepper to Taste

Directions:

Refrigerate all ingredients for three hours before serving.

Watercress & Blood Orange Salad

Servings: 4

Preparation Time: 10 Minutes

Calories: 94

Protein: 2 Grams

Fat: 5 Grams

Carbs: 13 Grams

Ingredients:

1 Tablespoon Hazelnuts, Toasted & Chopped

2 Blood Oranges (or Navel Oranges)

3 Cups watercress, Stems Removed

1/8 Teaspoon Sea Salt, Fine

1 Tablespoon Lemon Juice, Fresh

1 Tablespoon Honey, Raw

1 Tablespoon Water

2 Tablespoons Chives, Fresh

Directions:

Whisk your oil, honey, lemon juice, chives, salt and water together. Add in your watercress, tossing until it's coated.

Arrange the mixture onto salad plates, and top with orange slices. Drizzle with remaining liquid, and sprinkle with hazelnuts.

Parsley Salad

Servings: 8

Preparation Time: 30 Minutes

Calories: 165.2

Protein: 3.8 Grams

Fat: 9.1 Grams

Carbs: 20.1 Grams

Ingredients:

3 Lemons, Juiced

150 Grams Flat Lea Parsley, Chopped Fine

1 Cup Boiled Water

5 Tablespoons Olive Oil

Sea Salt & Black Pepper to Taste

6 Green Onions, Chopped Fine

1 Cup Bulgur

4 Tomatoes, Chopped Fine

Directions:

Add your Bulgur to your water, and mix well. Put a towel on top of it to steam it. Keep it to the side, and then chop your spring onions, tomatoes and parsley. Put them in your salad bowl.

Pour your juice into the mixture, and then add in your olive oil, salt and pepper.

Put this mixture over your bulgur to serve.

Tomato Eggplant Spinach Salad

Preparation Time: 30 minutes

Servings: 4

Calories: 163

Fat: 13 g

Carbohydrates: 10 g

Sugar: 3 g

Protein 2 g

Cholesterol: 0 mg

Ingredients:

1 large eggplant, cut into 3/4 inch slices

5 oz spinach

1 tbsp sun-dried tomatoes, chopped

1 tbsp oregano, chopped

1 tbsp parsley, chopped

1 tbsp fresh mint, chopped

1 tbsp shallot, chopped

For dressing:

1/4 cup olive oil

1/2 lemon juice

1/2 tsp smoked paprika

1 tsp Dijon mustard

1 tsp tahini

2 garlic cloves, minced

Pepper

Salt

Directions:

Place sliced eggplants into the large bowl and sprinkle with salt and set aside for minutes.

In a small bowl mix together all dressing ingredients. Set aside.

Heat grill to medium-high heat.

In a large bowl, add shallot, sun-dried tomatoes, herbs, and spinach.

Rinse eggplant slices and pat dry with paper towel.

Brush eggplant slices with olive oil and grill on medium high heat for 3-4 minutes on each side.

Let cool the grilled eggplant slices then cut into quarters.

Add eggplant to the salad bowl and pour dressing over salad. Toss well.

Serve and enjoy.

Cauliflower Radish Salad

Preparation Time: 15 minutes

Servings: 4

Calories: 58

Fat: 3.8 g

Carbohydrates: 5.6 g

Sugar: 2.1 g

Protein: 2.1 g

Cholesterol: 0 mg

Ingredients:

12 radishes, trimmed and chopped

1 tsp dried dill

1 tsp Dijon mustard

1 tbsp cider vinegar

1 tbsp olive oil

1 cup parsley, chopped

½ medium cauliflower head, trimmed and chopped

½ tsp black pepper

¼ tsp sea salt

Directions:

In a mixing bowl, combine together cauliflower, parsley, and radishes.

In a small bowl, whisk together olive oil, dill, mustard, vinegar, pepper, and salt.

Pour dressing over salad and toss well.

Serve immediately and enjoy.

Celery Salad

Preparation Time: 10 minutes

Servings: 6

Calories: 38

 Fat: 2.5 g

Carbohydrates: 3.3 g

Sugar: 1.5 g

 Protein: 0.8 g

Cholesterol 0 mg

Ingredients:

 6 cups celery, sliced

¼ tsp celery seed

1 tbsp lemon juice

2 tsp lemon zest, grated

1 tbsp parsley, chopped

1 tbsp olive oil

Sea salt

Directions:

Add all ingredients into the large mixing bowl and toss well.

Serve immediately and enjoy.

Chapter 6. Desserts & Snacks

Lemon Raspberry Fat Bombs

Preparation time: 10 minutes

Cooking time: 0 minutes

Servings: 12

Ingredients

1 ½ cups of boiled water

1 cup raw cashews

1 cup coconut, shredded

¼ cup of coconut oil

2 tablespoons sugar

½ teaspoon lemon zest

1 tablespoon lemon juice

1 cup raspberries

Directions:

Layer a muffin tray with paper cups and set it aside.

Now blend all other ingredients (except raspberries) in a blender.

Divide half of the batter into the muffin cups.

Add raspberries to the remaining batter in the blender.

Blend again then divide the berries batter into the muffin cups.

Freeze the muffin cups for 4 hours in the freezer.

Serve.

Nutrition:

Calories: 398

Total Fat: 6 g

Saturated Fat: 7 g

Cholesterol: 632 mg

Sodium: 497 mg

Total Carbs: 91 g

Fiber: 3 g

Sugar: 83 g

Protein: 2 g

Crunchy Chocolate Brownies

Preparation time: 10 minutes

Cooking time: 2 minutes

Servings: 10

Ingredients

Filling

2 cups dates, pitted

2 cups walnuts

¾ cup raw cacao

Pinch of sea salt

2 tablespoons water, added gradually

Topping

1 dark chocolate bar, chopped

½ cup peanut butter

1 tablespoon coconut oil

Directions:

Soak the pitted dates in water for 10 minutes, then drain.

Add walnuts to a blender and pulse until it forms a crumble.

Stir sea salt, cacao powder, dates, and 1 tablespoon water into the blender.

Blend again until it forms a thick date dough.

Spread this mixture in an 8-inch baking pan, lined with parchment sheet.

Press the dough in the pan then freeze for 1 hour.

Meanwhile, melt peanut butter, coconut oil, and chocolate chips in a glass bowl by heating in the microwave.

Pour this chocolate melt over the dates batter.

Allow it to sit, then slice.

Serve.

Nutrition:

Calories: 232

Total Fat: 8.9 g

Saturated Fat: 4.5 g

Cholesterol: 57 mg

Sodium: 340 mg

Total Carbs: 24.7 g

Fiber: 1.2 g

Sugar: 12.3 g

Protein: 5.3 g

Peanut Butter Chocolate Cups

Preparation time: 10 minutes

Cooking time: 3 minutes

Servings: 12

Ingredients

1 ½ cups vegan chocolate chips

¼ cup peanut butter

Directions:

Add peanut butter to a glass bowl and melt it by heating in the microwave for 1 minute.

Divide it in a muffin tray lined with muffin cups.

Now melt the chocolate chips in a bowl by heating in the microwave for 2 minutes.

Divide the chocolate melt into the muffin cups, then freeze the tray for 2 hours.

Serve the peanut butter chocolate cups.

Nutrition:

Calories: 427

Total Fat: 31.1 g

Saturated Fat: 4.2 g

Cholesterol: 123 mg

Sodium: 86 mg

Total Carbs: 9 g

Sugar: 12.4 g

Fiber: 19.8 g

Protein: 3.5 g

Strawberry Cheesecake Bites

Preparation time: 10 minutes
Cooking time: 0 minutes
Servings: 12
Ingredients
Crust
1 cup pecans
6 Medjool dates, pitted
¼ cup coconut, shredded
¼ teaspoon sea salt
Filling
1 cup raw cashews, soaked
¼ cup agave nectar
 2 tablespoons lemon juice
½ cup frozen strawberry slices
¼ cup coconut oil, melted
Topping
½ cup frozen strawberries, sliced
Directions:
Soak the dates in warm water for 10 minutes then drain.
Transfer the dates to a blender along with all other ingredients for the crust.
Blend until it forms a crumbly mixture tray with a muffin cup.
Line 2–12 muffin cups
Spread 1 ½ teaspoons of the mixture at the bottom of each muffin cup in a muffin tray.
Blend drained cashews, strawberry slices, coconut oil, lemon juice, and agave nectar in the blender.
Divide the filling into the muffin cups and freeze for 2 hours.
Garnish with the strawberries.
Serve.
Nutrition:
Calories: 398
Total Fat: 13.8 g
Saturated Fat: 5.1 g
Cholesterol: 200 mg
Sodium: 272 mg
Total Carbs: 53.6 g
Fiber: 1 g
Sugar: 12.3 g
Protein: 1.8 g

Chickpea Meringues

Preparation time: 10 minutes

Cooking time: 2 hours

Servings: 12

Ingredients

1 (15 oz) can chickpeas

¼ teaspoon cream of tartar

Kosher salt

¾ cup of sugar

Directions:

Layer 2 baking sheets with parchment paper and preheat the oven to 250°F.

Drain the chickpeas and reserve ¾ cup of its liquid.

Blend the chickpeas with cream of tartar, a pinch of salt, and the reserved liquid in the blender.

Add this mixture to a piping bag and pipe the mixture drop by drop onto the baking sheet.

Bake the meringue drops for 2 hours in the preheated oven.

Serve.

Nutrition:

Calories: 265

Total Fat: 14 g

Saturated Fat: 7 g

Cholesterol: 632 mg

Sodium: 497 mg

Total Carbs: 6 g

Fiber: 3 g

Sugar: 10 g

Protein: 5 g

Spinach and Artichoke Dip

Preparation time: 10 minutes

Cooking time: 14 minutes

Servings: 12

Ingredients

1 cup vegetable broth

1 lb cauliflower, cored and cut into florets

2 oz raw cashews

¼ cup vegan mayonnaise

2 tablespoons nutritional yeast

1 tablespoon Dijon mustard

1 tablespoon fresh lemon juice

2 teaspoons garlic powder

Kosher salt

2 large garlic cloves, minced

2 tablespoons olive oil

1 (10 oz) box frozen spinach, thawed

1 (14 oz) can artichokes, drained and halved

Freshly ground black pepper

Directions:

Preheat the oven to 350°F.

Place a deep skillet over medium heat and add vegetable stock.

Cook the stock to a simmer then add cauliflower and cashews.

Cover the cauliflower and cook for 10 minutes, or until its tender.

Puree this mixture with the help of a handheld blender for 1 minute.

Stir in yeast, mayonnaise, lemon juice, mustard, salt, and garlic powder.

Mix well and set the cauliflower blend aside.

Sauté garlic with olive oil in a skillet over medium heat for 2 minutes.

Stir in spinach, and a pinch of salt, then sauté for 1 minute.

Transfer this spinach mixture to a blender along with artichokes.

Blender these veggies until smooth, then add salt and black pepper.

Mix well, then add the cauliflower mixture.

Spread the artichoke dip in a casserole dish then broil for 1 minute in the oven.

Serve with chips.

Nutrition:

Calories: 172

Total Fat: 11.8 g

Saturated Fat: 4.4 g

Cholesterol: 62 mg

Sodium: 871 mg

Total Carbs: 45.8 g

Fiber: 0.6 g

Sugar: 2.3 g

Protein: 4 g

Malt Glazed Wheat Thins

Preparation time: 10 minutes

Cooking time: 12 minutes

Servings: 12

Ingredients

Glaze

2 oz light corn syrup

¼ oz barley malt syrup

¼ teaspoon kosher salt

1 oz hot water

Crackers

5 oz whole wheat flour

2 ½ oz sugar

1 ½ oz bread flour

¾ oz toasted wheat germ

½ teaspoon ground turmeric

½ teaspoon kosher salt

½ teaspoon cream of tartar

¼ teaspoon baking soda

1 oz coconut oil

¼ oz barley malt syrup

3 oz water

Directions:

Prepare the glaze by mixing corn syrup with salt and barley syrup in a small bowl.

Stir in hot water while mixing it continuously, then set it aside.

Now place the oven rack in the lower middle portion and preheat it for 350°F.

Mix wheat flour with bread flour, sugar, wheat germ, cream of tartar, turmeric, salt, coconut oil, and baking soda in a blender.

Mix barley malt with water then add to the flour mixture.

Knead this mixture well to form a dough.

Layer a baking sheet with a parchment sheet.

Roll the dough on a floured surface into a 5x8 inch rectangle and 1/16-inch thick.

Place the flour sheet on the parchment sheet and spread the prepared glaze on its top.

Slice the dough sheet into 1 ½-inch squares.

Bake the dough for 12 minutes, or until crispy.

Serve.

Nutrition:

Calories: 246

Total Fat: 7.4 g

Saturated Fat: 4.6 g

Cholesterol: 105 mg

Sodium: 353 mg

Total Carbs: 29.4 g

Sugar: 6.5 g

Fiber: 2.7 g

Protein: 7.2 g

Potato Chips with Thyme

Preparation time: 10 minutes

Cooking time: 13 minutes

Servings: 12

Ingredients

3 tablespoons nutritional yeast

¼ oz dried mushrooms

¼ teaspoon lemon zest

¼ teaspoon garlic, minced

1 teaspoon fresh thyme, minced

 4 potatoes, sliced thinly

Kosher salt and ground black pepper, to taste

Directions:

Add dried mushrooms, lemon zest, garlic powder, thyme, and yeast to a blender and blend well.

Toss the potatoes slices with this mixture onto a baking sheet.

Bake the slices for 8 minutes at 350°F, then toss them well.

Continue baking for another 5 minutes.

Serve.

Nutrition:

Calories: 293

Total Fat: 16 g

Saturated Fat: 2.3 g

Cholesterol: 75 mg

Sodium: 386 mg

Total Carbs: 25.2 g

Sugar: 2.6 g

Fiber: 1.9 g

Protein: 4.2 g

Tofu Spring Rolls

Preparation time: 10 minutes

Cooking time: 10 minutes

Servings: 10

Ingredients

1 (14 oz) block firm tofu

3 tablespoons vegetable oil

¼ cup peanut tamarind sauce

1 large carrot, peeled and julienned

4 oz green peas

2 cups mixed fresh herbs

1 tablespoon toasted peanuts, chopped

20 dried spring roll rice paper wrappers

Directions:

Soak tofu in boiling water and strain in the colander for 1 minute.

Place a non-stick skillet over medium heat and add vegetable oil.

Pat the tofu dry and slice into 2-inch-long thick sticks.

Add the tofu to the hot oil and sear it for 10 minutes until golden-brown on all sides.

Toss the seared tofu with peanut tamarind sauce in a large bowl.

Mix the tofu with carrots, greens, peppers, herbs, and peanuts in a large bowl.

Spread the rice wrappers on a working surface and divide the tofu filling into the wrappers.

Wrap the rice paper around the tofu filling.

Serve.

Nutrition:

Calories: 319

Total Fat: 10.6 g

Saturated Fat: 3.1 g

Cholesterol: 131 mg

Sodium: 834 mg

Total Carbs: 31.4 g

Fiber: 0.2 g

Sugar: 0.3 g

Protein: 4.6 g

Sicilian Eggplant Caponata

Preparation time: 10 minutes

Cooking time: 8 minutes

Servings: 4

Ingredients

1 cup pine nuts

½ cup olive oil

1 small globe eggplant, cut into ¾-inch dice

Kosher salt and ground black pepper, to taste

4 scallions, white parts only, sliced

1 rib celery, diced

1 red bell pepper, diced

4 garlic cloves, sliced

2 tablespoons fresh mint leaves

2 tablespoons parsley leaves, minced

2 tablespoons tomato paste

½ teaspoon ground cinnamon

½ cup raisins

2 tablespoons capers, drained and rinsed

2 tablespoons sugar

2 tablespoons red wine vinegar

2 tablespoons balsamic vinegar

Directions:

Place a large pan over medium heat and add 1 teaspoon olive oil and half of pine nuts.

Stir them for 2 minutes then transfer them to a bowl.

Add 4 tablespoons oil to the same pan, and add eggplant to sauté for 6 minutes.

Add bell pepper, garlic, celery, and scallions, then stir for 3 minutes.

Toss in remaining pine nuts, parsley, mint, parsley, cinnamon, tomato paste, sugar, raisins, capers, balsamic vinegar, remaining olive oil, and red wine vinegar.

Bring this mixture to a simmer and adjust seasoning with salt and black pepper.

Serve.

Nutrition:

Calories: 211

Total Fat: 25.5 g

Saturated Fat: 12.4 g

Cholesterol: 69 mg

Sodium: 58 mg

Total Carbs: 32.4 g

Fiber: 0.7 g

Sugar: 0.3 g

Protein: 1.4 g

Conclusion

There are so many powerful and persuasive reasons to make a positive change and switch over to a plant-based diet. A plant-based diet will improve your quality of life, give you more energy and vitality, help you lose unwanted body fat, and it may even lengthen your years on this beautiful planet. As a bonus, by making the change you will be making a real and significant difference to our planet Earth's future. So much energy and fossil fuels are wasted by sourcing meat and other animal products, transporting them from place to place across miles and miles of road, and processing all of these animal products.

On top of that, there is an enormous crisis of animals being treated extremely inhumanely and cruelly. In order to mass produce meat and animal products to meet the enormous demand of the market, many manufacturers put animal comfort and quality of life last and do not make it a priority to treat them in a humane and ethical fashion.

There is also an incredible amount of food waste that happens in the production and processing of animal products. Extraordinary amounts of energy and resources are expended and too much gets simply thrown away. By switching to a plant-based diet, you will be greatly decreasing your carbon footprint and ensuring that fewer animals have to suffer at the hands of humans. And isn't that a good feeling?

Considering all the ethical reasons for switching to a plant-based diet, the enormous health benefits and improved quality of life are the icing on an already extremely appealing cake. Eating real food that grows from earth is the most important thing. Most likely, the reason people don't eat enough plant-based food is that they still don't realize how strong plant nutrients are in maintaining our health.

Most people still feed on the flesh and products of other animals, not because there is something so natural, necessary or rational about it, but primarily because the major marketing share in supermarkets, stores, and food advertising are occupied by meat, animal, fast, processed and packaged products. Vegetable foods without salt, sugar, and refined fat still account for only a small percentage of the food industry's profits.

Follow my plant-based diet meal plan and be ready to cook some amazing recipes that can help you to stay healthy.

Wish you good luck with plant-based diet!

www.ingramcontent.com/pod-product-compliance
Lightning Source LLC
Chambersburg PA
CBHW081305250726

48662CB00008B/2411